HANDBOOK OF CRITICAL CARE PROCEDURES AND THERAPY

Handbook of Critical Care Procedures and Therapy

Roy D. Cane, M.B.B.Ch., F.F.A. (S.A.)
Professor of Anesthesiology
University of South Florida College of Medicine
Tampa, Florida

Richard Davison, M.D.
Associate Professor of Medicine
Northwestern University Medical School
Chicago, Illinois

Michael H. Albrink, M.D.
Assistant Professor of Surgery
University of South Florida College of Medicine
Tampa, Florida

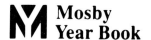

Mosby
Year Book

St. Louis   Baltimore   Boston   Chicago   London   Philadelphia   Sydney   Toronto

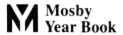
Mosby
Year Book

Dedicated to Publishing Excellence

Sponsoring Editor: Susan M. Gay
Assistant Editor: Sandra E. Clark
Assistant Director, Manuscript Services: Frances M. Perveiler
Production Supervisor: Karen Halm
Proofroom Manager: Barbara Kelly

Mosby–Year Book, Inc.
11830 Westline Industrial Drive
St. Louis, MO 63146

1 2 3 4 5 6 7 8 9 0 CL DC 96 95 94 93 92

Library of Congress Cataloging-in-Publication Data
Handbook of critical care procedures and therapy / [edited by] Roy
   D. Cane, Richard Davison, Michael H. Albrink.
       p.   cm.
   Includes bibliographical references and index.
   ISBN 0-8016-6555-8
   1. Critical care medicine. 2. Surgical emergencies. I. Cane,
Roy D. II. Davison, Richard, 1937- . III. Albrink, Michael H.
   [DNLM: 1. Critical Care—methods—handbooks. WX 39
H233]
   RC86.7.H364 1992
   616'.028—dc20   92-12915
   DNLM/DLC   CIP
   for Library of Congress

We dedicate this book to all academic physicians who, by teaching and example, help to perpetuate the art and science of the practice of critical care medicine. In particular we acknowledge the contribution of our own "special" teachers:

Barry A. Shapiro, M.D.
(R.D.C.)

Lisette Glusberg, M.D.
(R.D.)

Karen Wells, M.D. & Kelly
(M.H.A.)

CONTRIBUTORS

Michael H. Albrink, M.D.
Assistant Professor
   of Surgery
University of South Florida
   College of Medicine
Tampa, Florida

**Roy D. Cane, M.B.B.Ch.,
F.F.A. (S.A.)**
Professor of Anesthesiology
University of South Florida
   College of Medicine
Tampa, Florida

Joan M. Christie, M.D.
Assistant Professor
   of Anesthesiology
University of South Florida
   College of Medicine
Tampa, Florida

Robert M. Craig, M.D.
Associate Professor
   of Medicine
Northwestern University
   Medical School
Chicago, Illinois

Daniel J. Fintel, M.D.
Assistant Professor
   of Medicine
Northwestern University
   Medical School
Chicago, Illinois

Thomas G. Frolich, M.D.
Assistant Professor
   of Clinical Medicine
Northwestern University
   Medical School
Chicago, Illinois

Daniel R. Ganger, M.D.
Assistant Professor
   of Clinical Medicine
Northwestern University
   Medical School
Chicago, Illinois

Jeffrey Goldberger, M.D.
Assistant Professor
   of Medicine
Northwestern University
   Medical School
Chicago, Illinois

**Michael D. Hammond,
M.D.**
Associate Professor
   of Medicine
University of South Florida
   College of Medicine
Tampa, Florida

Robert C. Hendel, M.D.
Assistant Professor
   of Medicine
Northwestern University
   Medical School
Chicago, Illinois

Kenneth L. Holling, M.D.
Fellow in Pulmonary
  and Critical Care Medicine
University of South Florida
  College of Medicine
Tampa, Florida

Debra L. Isaac, B.N., M.D.
Fellow in Cardiology
Northwestern University
  Medical School
Chicago, Illinois

Michael T. Johnson, D.O.
Instructor in Anesthesiology
University of South Florida
  College of Medicine
Tampa, Florida

Alan Kadish, M.D.
Associate Professor
  of Medicine
Northwestern University
  Medical School
Chicago, Illinois

Susan Markowsky, Pharm.D.
Assistant Professor
  of Clinical Anesthesiology
University of South Florida
  College of Medicine
Tampa, Florida

Richard A. Pomerantz, M.D.
Assistant Professor
  of Clinical Surgery
Northwestern University
  Medical School
Chicago, Illinois

Jukka Räsänen, M.D.
Associate Professor
  of Anesthesiology
University of South Florida
  College of Medicine
Tampa, Florida

Carl L. Tommaso, M.D.
Associate Professor
  of Medicine
Northwestern University
  Medical School
Chicago, Illinois

PREFACE

The practice of critical care medicine includes invasive diagnostic and monitoring interventions and mechanical supportive therapy. These interventions and therapies are associated with the potential for significant complications and physiologic disadvantages. The critical care practitioner frequently is required to assess the relative risk:benefit relationship of the use of a given modality of diagnosis, monitoring, or therapy. Use of consistent, careful techniques in the application of these interventions and therapies can help to reduce the risk of complications and improve patient outcome. The techniques described in this book, while by no means the only way to implement a particular modality, are all tried and tested methods that have been safely employed by the authors in the management of a large number of critically ill patients.

The topics chosen represent procedures commonly indicated in the management of a wide range of critically ill, adult medical and surgical patients. We chose not to include procedures used in the management of critically ill pediatric patients because pediatric critical care is a discipline with unique features. The first three chapters describe techniques for invasive hemodynamic monitoring. The second section (Chapters 4 through 10) includes techniques usually used to facilitate diagnosis. The final section of the book (Chapters 11 through 29) describes techniques for the provision of supportive therapy. The information included in each chapter is not intended to be a comprehensive discussion of available knowledge on that topic. Rather, we have attempted to provide the clinician with sufficient information to perform a given procedure safely. Readers are urged to supplement this text with further reading, hence, the "Suggested Reading" section at the end of every chapter.

We wish to acknowledge the contribution to our knowledge and understanding made by all the students, residents, and fellows we have been privileged to teach. We thank the contributing authors for their chapters and patience with our editorial suggestions. Thanks are due to our colleagues for their support and understanding, in particular Drs. John Downs, Larry Carey, Jukka Räsänen, Joan Christie, Michael Johnson, Alexander Rosemurgy, Daniel Fintel, and Robert Hendel. We acknowledge and thank Terry McBride, Lois Pomerantz, and Margo McKnight for the artwork, Davey Volkhardt and Valerie Fumea for editorial assistance, and Xenia Ruiz and Rosemarie Klimley for secretarial assistance. A special thank you is owed to Millie Casanova, without whose untiring labor, unfailing enthusiasm, and dedication this manuscript would not have been completed.

Roy D. Cane, M.B.B.Ch., F.F.A. (S.A.)
Richard Davison, M.D.
Michael H. Albrink, M.D.

CONTENTS

1

Arterial Catheterization

Roy D. Cane, M.B.B.Ch., F.F.A.(S.A.)

INTRODUCTION

Cannulation of a peripheral artery is a frequently employed, safe technique for arterial pressure monitoring and blood gas sampling in critically ill patients.

OBJECTIVE

To place and secure in an indwelling catheter in a peripheral artery.

Indications

1. Continuous arterial pressure monitoring.
2. Frequent arterial blood sampling.

Contraindications

1. Inadequate collateral flow.
2. Peripheral vascular disease.

PREPARATION

Choice of Artery

Arterial puncture and cannulation may be associated with vessel spasm, intraluminal clotting, or periarterial bleeding and hematoma formation. These factors may result in diminution or interruption of blood flow to the tissues supplied by that artery. Therefore, adequate collateral blood flow is an **essential** consideration when choosing a site for arterial cannulation. The arteries of the hands (radial and ulnar arteries) and feet (dorsalis pedis artery) usually have good collateral flow. Collateral flow around the brachial artery is adequate. The femoral artery has poor collateral flow below the inguinal ligament. Generally, superficial arteries are easier to palpate, stabilize, and puncture. With these factors in mind, the recommended sites for arterial cannulation, in order of descending preference, are

1. Radial artery.
2. Brachial artery.
3. Dorsalis pedis artery.

Ensuring that the collateral flow to the hand from the ulnar artery is adequate **before** placing a catheter in the radial artery is **mandatory.** Failure to do so may result in ischemia to the digits and possible gangrene.

Determination of the Adequacy of Ulnar Artery Collateral Flow

Arterial blood supply to the digits of the hand arises from the superficial palmar arch formed by anastomosis of the radial and ulnar arteries. Normally, the dominant blood supply comes from the ulnar artery; however, radial artery dominance is not uncommon, and an interrupted superficial palmar arch is occasionally present. Two techniques are available for the bedside determination of the adequacy of ulnar artery collateral flow to the digits:

1. Modified Allen's test.
2. Digital pulse plethysmography.

Modified Allen's Test

This technique (Fig 1–1) is the traditionally recommended method of demonstrating the adequacy of flow from the ulnar artery to the hand and fingers. The patient's hand is closed tightly to form a fist; thus, the blood is forced from the hand. Pressure is applied directly at the wrist to compress and obstruct *both* the radial and ulnar arteries. The hand is then relaxed but not fully extended, revealing a blanched palm and fingers. The obstructing pressure is removed from **only** the ulnar artery, while the patient's palm, fingers, and thumb are observed. They should become flushed within 10 to 15 seconds as blood from the ulnar artery refills the empty capillary beds. A positive modified Allen's test confirms that the ulnar artery collateral flow is adequate and that placement of an indwelling catheter in the radial artery is safe. Failure to see the entire hand flush on release of the ulnar artery is considered a negative modified Allen's test and is associated with either radial artery dominant flow to the hand or an interrupted superficial palmar arch. **Following a negative modified Allen's test, the radial artery should not be cannulated under any circumstances.**

If the patient cannot make a fist, or flushing of the hand on release of the ulnar artery is not clearly seen, digital pulse plethysmography offers an alternative technique for determining which artery provides the dominant flow to the hand. If the modified Allen's test is equivocal, an attempt to define the dominant flow to the hand with digital pulse plethysmography is essential before attempting arterial cannulation.

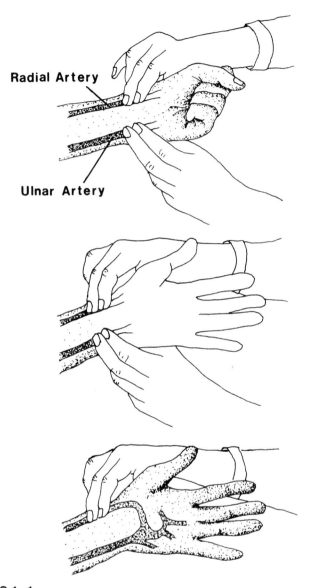

Radial Artery

Ulnar Artery

FIG 1–1.
Modified Allen's test. **Top,** the hand is clenched into a tight fist and the radial and ulnar arteries are compressed. **Middle,** the hand is opened, the palm and fingers appear blanched. **Bottom,** on release of compression of the ulnar artery, flushing of the hand is noted. (From Shapiro BA et al: Guidelines for obtaining blood gas samples, in *Clinical application of blood gases,* ed 4, St. Louis, 1989, Mosby–Year Book, p 252. Used by permission.)

Digital Pulse Plethysmography

This technique requires use of a pulse oximeter with a visual display of the arterial pulse waveform.

1. Place the pulse oximeter sensor on the patient's index finger and observe a trace of the pulse waveform and amplitude.
2. Compress the radial artery and observe the pulse wave tracing. Two things may happen.
   a. The pulse waveform and amplitude will *not change*, indicating that the dominant arterial supply is from the ulnar artery (Fig 1–2). To confirm this finding, with the pulse oximeter sensor still on the index finger, release the radial artery compression, and then compress the ulnar artery. If the dominant flow is from the ulnar artery, you will see a change in waveform and amplitude (Fig 1–3).

ULNAR DOMINANT SUPPLY

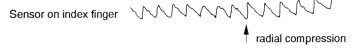

Sensor on index finger

↑ radial compression

FIG 1–2.
Pulse plethysmographic tracing with radial artery compression and dominant blood supply from the ulnar artery.

ULNAR DOMINANT SUPPLY

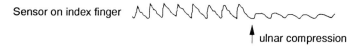

Sensor on index finger

↑ ulnar compression

FIG 1–3.
Pulse plethysmographic tracing with ulnar artery compression and dominant blood flow from the ulnar artery.

   b. The pulse waveform and amplitude will *change* (Fig 1–4), indicating that the dominant flow is from the radial artery, or that the patient has an interrupted superficial palmar arch.

RADIAL DOMINANT SUPPLY

Sensor on index finger

↑ radial compression

FIG 1−4.
Pulse plethysmographic tracing with radial artery compression and dominant blood flow from the radial artery.

3. To differentiate between radial artery dominant flow or an interrupted superficial palmar arch, place the pulse oximeter sensor on the patient's fourth finger and note the waveform and amplitude. Compression of the ulnar artery will effect no change in the waveform and amplitude (Fig 1−5) if the dominant flow is from the radial artery.

RADIAL DOMINANT SUPPLY

Sensor on 4th finger

↑ ulnar compression

FIG 1−5.
Pulse plethysmographic tracing with ulnar artery compression and dominant blood flow from the radial artery.

If the pulse waveform and amplitude are diminished following ulnar artery compression (Fig 1−6), an interrupted superficial palmar arch exists.

INTERRUPTED SUPERFICIAL PALMER ARCH

Sensor on 4th finger

↑ ulnar compression

FIG 1−6.
Pulse plethysmographic tracing with ulnar artery compression and blood flow through an interrupted superficial palmar arch.

If the dominant flow to the hand is from the ulnar artery, proceed with the radial artery cannulation. If the dominant flow is from the radial artery, or if the patient has an interrupted superficial palmar arch, **do not** cannulate either radial or ulnar artery. Instead, attempt to cannulate the dorsalis pedis or brachial artery.

Equipment

1. Twenty-gauge intravascular catheter with central stylet.
2. Iodophor and alcohol swabs.
3. Three-milliliter syringe of 1% lidocaine with a 25-gauge needle.
4. Tape.
5. Arterial line flushing assembly (provided by nursing staff).

Required Monitoring

Required Laboratory Data

Coagulation profile, including prothrombin time, partial thromboplastin time, and platelet count.

PROCEDURE (Fig 1−7)

1. Introduce yourself to the patient; explain why the procedure is necessary, and what you are about to do.
2. Perform a modified Allen's test or digital pulse plethysmography to determine the dominant blood flow to the hand. If the patient has ulnar artery dominance, proceed with radial artery cannulation. If radial artery cannulation is contraindicated, attempt dorsalis pedis or brachial artery cannulation.
3. Put on sterile gloves.
4. Clean the skin over the puncture site with iodophor and then with alcohol.
5. Raise a skin weal with the 1% lidocaine through the 25-gauge needle.

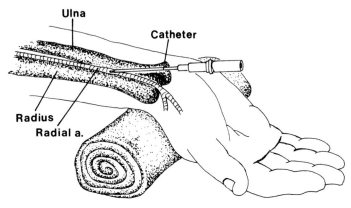

FIG 1–7.
Catheter insertion in the radial artery. Position and stabilize the arm with the wrist extended. Note that the catheter enters the artery at an acute angle to the skin.

6. With the patient's wrist cocked, place two or three fingers of your left/right hand over the maximal pulsation of the radial artery, proximal to the selected puncture site, to stabilize the vessel and define its long axis.

7. With the intravascular catheter held in your other hand, penetrate the skin over the pulse at a narrow angle to the skin. Advance the catheter until blood exits the hub of the catheter. (Some clinicians prefer to advance the catheter rapidly to transfix the artery and then to withdraw it slowly until blood exits the hub.) Once blood is flowing out of the catheter hub, hold the hub and stylet steady with one hand and advance the catheter over the stylet up the artery. If the catheter does not slide freely, remove the entire catheter and stylet from the patient's skin, compress the puncture site to prevent hematoma formation, and reattempt the procedure. **Never** introduce the stylet into the catheter when the catheter is in the patient's skin. You may cut off the tip of the catheter, which may then be embolized to a terminal branch of the artery.

8. Connect the catheter to the arterial line flushing assembly and tape securely. Cover the site with a bacteria-impermeable, transparent dressing. Connect the

arterial line flushing assembly to the previously calibrated bedside pressure monitor.

9. Examine the pulse waveform to verify that an artery has been cannulated.

FOLLOW-UP

1. Daily, inspect the site for evidence of infection (edema, erythema, exudation). If the site appears infected, immediately remove the catheter and send the tip to the bacteriology laboratory for culture. If an arterial cannula is still required for the management of the patient, establish a fresh cannula in another site.

2. If the cannula is kinked or partially obstructed, as manifested by an abnormal, or damped pulse waveform, replace it with a fresh cannula. The original site can be reused if it is clean.

COMPLICATIONS

1. *Diminished or temporarily absent arterial flow.* An incidence of between 7% and 41% has been reported with ultrasound flow studies. If collateral flow is adequate, a diminished or absent flow will not result in patient morbidity. With inadequate collateral flow, necrosis and tissue loss have been reported, including loss of fingers and toes. Lower limb loss following femoral artery cannulation has also been reported.

2. *Thrombosis.* The incidence of radial artery thrombosis can be reduced by proper cannulation techniques and preadministration of aspirin.

3. *Infection.* Both local and systemic infections may occur. Infection rates for arterial cannulas that are placed and maintained with the proper aseptic technique are similar to infection rates for venous catheters.

4. *False arterial pressure readings.* Falsely elevated ar-

terial pressure readings have been reported with the automatic flushing devices.

DOCUMENTATION

Documentation should include the following:

1. Indication for arterial cannulation.
2. Choice of site of cannulation. If the radial artery was used, indicate the technique that was used to verify collateral flow to the hand. If the radial artery was not used, provide justification for choice of an alternative site.
3. Size and type of catheter used.
4. Complications encountered, if any.
5. Adequacy of pulse waveform, initial blood pressure readings, and initial arterial blood gas results obtained from arterial catheter.

SUGGESTED READING

Fragen RJ: Arterial catheterization and maintenance of indwelling arterial lines. In Beal JM, editor: *Critical care for surgical patients*, New York, 1982, Macmillan, pp 91–101.

Shapiro BA et al: *Clinical application of blood gases*, ed 4, St Louis, 1989, Mosby–Year Book, pp 248–258.

2

Central Venous Catheterization

Richard A. Pomerantz, M.D.

INTRODUCTION

Infraclavicular subclavian vein catheterization was described in 1952 and became a popular procedure in the 1960s. Catheterization of the internal jugular vein was popularized in the late 1960s. Central venous catheterization has become a routine procedure, particularly in the critical care setting, as the number of applications has multiplied.

OBJECTIVE

Placement of a secure intravenous catheter in the central venous system.

Indications

1. Central venous pressure monitoring.
2. Access to the central venous system for the subsequent introduction of a pulmonary artery catheter.
3. Access for hypertonic parenteral nutritional support.

4. Access for administration of fluid and medications in the absence of peripheral venous access.

5. Hemodialysis.

Contraindications

1. Coagulopathy, thrombocytopenia, and prolonged bleeding time represent relative contraindications to subclavian venipuncture.

2. Central venous thrombosis.

3. Abnormal central venous anatomy.

4. Intravascular volume depletion is a relative contraindication.

PREPARATION

Choice of Central Venous Access Route

Either the subclavian or the internal jugular route is preferable to femoral vein catheterization. The site of access to the femoral vein at the groin is more susceptible to bacterial colonization and subsequent infection. Catheter stabilization at the femoral vein limits patient mobility more than at subclavian or internal jugular sites, and femoral vein thrombophlebitis is a potentially very morbid complication. Nevertheless, the femoral vein at the groin is readily accessible. Puncture and catheterization may be performed rapidly and safely, so that femoral venous access is an acceptable alternative.

The choice of subclavian versus internal jugular venous catheterization is a matter of preference. A catheter inserted below the clavicle into the subclavian vein is readily secured and allows for maximum patient mobility and comfort. However, the subclavian vein is not readily accessible to direct pressure should bleeding occur during insertion. Therefore, the presence of any form of a coagulopathy or an abnormality of platelet number or function represents a relative contraindication to subclavian venipuncture. Furthermore, the risk of iatrogenic pneumothorax is less with internal jugular vein catheterization in the neck.

When a documented coagulopathy or thrombocytopenia exists, cut-down at the cephalic vein in the deltopectoral groove or the basilar vein above the elbow is a reliable and safe alternative to direct puncture. With acute trauma, peripheral venous cut-down is a safer means of establishing intravenous access.

Choice of Catheter Design and Composition

A variety of central venous catheters are commercially available. Catheters differ in material composition, in the size and number of lumina, and in flow characteristics. The most commonly used materials are radiopaque polyurethane and silicone elastomer. Central venous catheters should be radiopaque. Catheter choice is based on a proved record of safety and durability and on the specific purpose for which it is required. Catheter materials differ in thrombogenicity and flexibility, which in part, determine potential complications. Soft, flexible, nonthrombogenic catheters are preferred.

Equipment

1. Preselected intravenous fluid with administration tubing.
2. Rolled towel.
3. Iodophor prep solution.
4. Mayo stand with sterile field.
5. Sterile towels.
6. Ten-milliliter syringe with Luer-Lok and 1.5-inch, 25-gauge needle for local anesthesia with 1% lidocaine.
7. Five-milliliter syringe, non-Luer-Lok.
8. Eighteen-gauge, 2.5-inch introducer needle.
9. Sterile Luer-Lok extension tubing.
10. Silk suture, 2-0, with cutting needle.
11. Disposable scalpel with number 11 blade.
12. Dual-purpose spring guidewire with a J-tip at

one end and straight soft tip at the other; 0.89-mm diameter, 60-cm length.

13. Vessel dilator.

14. Radiopaque 8-inch (20-cm) polyurethane catheter.

Required Monitoring

Monitoring of the patient with either a pulse oximeter or with continuous electrocardiographic tracing is appropriate, particularly for patients in the critical care setting. For patients outside critical care, the procedure may be performed at the bedside without monitoring. Femoral venous catheterization requires no specific monitoring.

Required Laboratory Data

1. Roentgenogram.

2. Prothrombin time, partial thromboplastin time, platelet count, and a bleeding time if clinically indicated.

PROCEDURE

Subclavian Venous Catheterization

1. In the elective setting, informed consent is indicated. Introduce yourself to the patient; explain the indications for the procedure, the procedure itself, and the potential complications. Answer questions the patient may have. Obtain written informed consent.

2. Ask the patient to assume a supine position. Place a rolled towel along the thoracic vertebral column between the scapulae, and ask the patient to allow his/her shoulders to fall back to the bed.

3. Wear operating room cap and mask, and ask your assistants to do the same.

4. Wash your hands.

5. Put on sterile gown and gloves.

6. Place the patient in 15° to 20° Trendelenburg; position yourself and your instruments on the side of the procedure, and prepare the field with iodophor solution. Isolate the field with sterile towels, providing yourself with a wide sterile field.

7. Palpate the appropriate anatomic landmarks (Fig 2–1). The site of infraclavicular subclavian venipuncture is the junction of the medial and middle thirds of the clavicle. The needle is directed toward the notch of the manubrium, parallel to the chest wall. Palpate the site of venipuncture with the index finger of the dominant hand and the notch of the manubrium with the index finger of the nondominant hand.

8. Infiltrate the site of venipuncture with 1% lidocaine with a 1.5-inch, 25-gauge needle. Create a dermal skin weal and then infiltrate the subcutaneous tissue down to and including the periosteum of the clavicle. Creating the skin weal approximately 2 cm lateral and 1 cm inferior to the junction of medial and middle thirds of the clavicle allows for a more gentle curve as the needle and catheter pass beneath the clavicle, thus lessening the risk that the catheter will kink at this point.

9. With the index finger of the nondominant hand on the notch of the manubrium as a guide to this land-

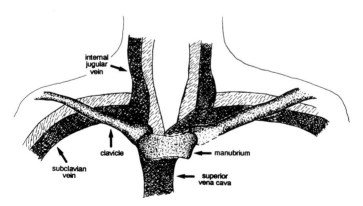

FIG 2–1.
Landmarks for subclavian venipuncture.

mark, use your dominant hand to pass a 2.5-inch, 18-gauge introducer needle on a 5-mL non-Luer-Lok syringe through the skin and subcutaneous tissue to the clavicle at junction of its medial and middle thirds (Fig 2–2). Keep the bevel of the needle directed caudally. Continue to pass the needle under the clavicle, aiming for the notch of the manubrium, with the trajectory of the needle parallel to the chest wall, while applying gentle suction on the syringe. A sudden rush of venous blood into the syringe indicates entry into the vein. Once blood return is obtained, advance the needle no farther. If no blood returns with passage of the needle, withdraw the needle while applying gentle suction to a point outside the clavicle. Then redirect slightly cephalad or slightly caudad, and make another pass. **Never redirect the needle without first withdrawing past the clavicle.** Lacerating the subclavian vein or artery by doing so is possible.

10. Once venipuncture is achieved, steady the needle with the nondominant hand; remove the syringe with a gentle twisting motion (use a non-Luer-Lok syringe); and place your thumb over the hub of the needle to prevent air from entering and blood from leaving (Fig 2–3). Ready the guidewire with the J-tip proximal. Ask the patient to take a deep breath and hold the breath.

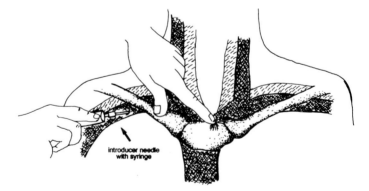

introducer needle
with syringe

FIG 2–2.
Infraclavicular subclavian venipuncture. Introducer needle passes under clavicle to reach the notch of the manubrium.

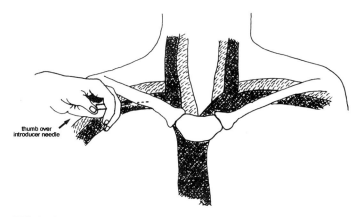

FIG 2–3.
Infraclavicular subclavian venipuncture. Thumb prevents air from entering the vein.

With the patient holding his/her breath, pass the guidewire through the needle and into the superior vena cava (Fig 2–4). Approximately 15 to 20 cm of the guidewire is required. The guidewire should pass easily, without resistance. Remove the needle from over the guidewire, and allow the patient to resume normal ventilation. If the guidewire does not pass easily, you may need to withdraw the needle 2 to 3 mm, as it is

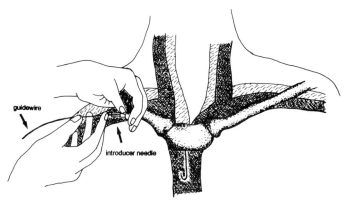

FIG 2–4.
Infraclavicular subclavian venipuncture—passage of guidewire.

possible for the needle to abut the back wall of the vein and prevent passage of the guidewire. If the guidewire will not pass after this simple maneuver, the introducer needle and guidewire should be withdrawn together, and another attempt made. **Never withdraw the guidewire through the needle.** The needle might shear off a portion of the guidewire, causing a foreign body embolus.

11. With the guidewire in place and the needle withdrawn, enlarge the cutaneous entry site with the disposable scalpel with a number 11 blade. Pass the vessel dilator over the guidewire into the subclavian vein to dilate the tract. Withdraw the vessel dilator only.

12. Pass the catheter over the guidewire into the subclavian vein and down into the superior vena cava. For the average-size adult, approximately 14 to 18 cm of catheter is required, as measured from the skin (Fig 2–5). Remove the guidewire and place the thumb of the nondominant hand over the hub of the catheter. Attach a 5-mL syringe to the catheter and aspirate venous blood. Doing so confirms intravascular placement of the catheter.

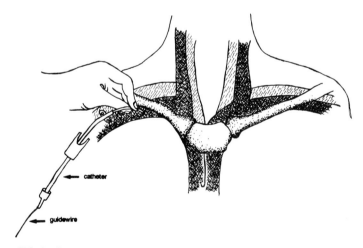

FIG 2–5.
Infraclavicular subclavian venipuncture—Seldinger catheter-over-guidewire technique.

When establishing central venous access with an introducer sheath, the vessel dilator may be passed through the introducer sheath, and then both passed over the guidewire. The guidewire is removed first, and subsequently the vessel dilator is removed, leaving the introducer sheath in place.

13. Attach the previously flushed Luer-Lok extension tubing from the intravenous fluid to the catheter and allow fluid to flush the line. Adjust the fluid rate to a minimum until radiographic confirmation of catheter placement. Secure the catheter with suture and cover with a sterile transparent adhesive dressing. Do not use antibiotic ointment at the catheter insertion site before applying the dressing.

14. Take the patient out of the Trendelenburg position and remove the rolled towel from behind the thoracic vertebral column.

Internal Jugular Venous Catheterization

1. Obtain written informed consent. Have all necessary materials, including intravenous (IV) fluid with tubing, ready before beginning.
2. Position the patient supine and place a rolled towel beneath the shoulders, allowing the patient's head to rest on the bed with the neck extended. Ask the patient to turn his/her head to the side opposite the procedure.
3. The procedure is performed from the head of the bed, requiring the headboard to be removed and the bed to be moved away from the wall to allow the operator room.
4. Wash, gown, and glove as for subclavian venous catheterization. Position the patient in the Trendelenburg position.
5. Prepare the operative site with iodophor solution and drape with sterile towels.
6. The internal jugular vein lies beneath the sternocleidomastoid muscle lateral and slightly anterior to the carotid artery (Fig 2–6). Palpation of

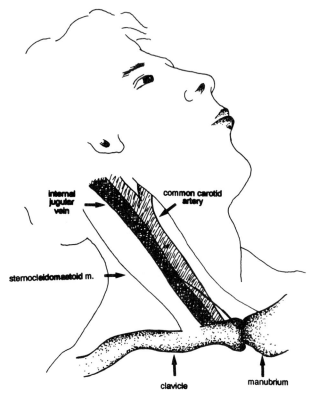

FIG 2–6.
Landmarks for internal jugular venipuncture.

the carotid artery pulse provides the landmark that localizes the internal jugular vein. Puncture and catheterization of the internal jugular vein may be approached anteriorly or posteriorly to the sternocleidomastoid muscle. The third option is to approach between the heads of the muscle slightly more caudad in the neck. The choice of puncture site is a matter of personal preference; however, it is important to keep the following in mind.

a. It is safest to approach the vein higher in the neck at approximately the level of the cricoid cartilage. This approach minimizes the risk of injury to the pleura.

    b. Furthermore, this approach avoids the risk of injury to the thoracic duct on the left. Catheterization of the right side will minimize the frequency of catheter malposition.

7. Infiltrate the puncture site with 1% lidocaine using a 1.5-inch, 25-gauge needle. Locate the vein with a 1.5-inch, 22-gauge seeker needle on a 5-mL non-Luer-Lok syringe. Palpate the carotid artery with the index and middle fingers of the nondominant hand. Pass the needle to a position immediately lateral to the carotid pulse, immediately deep to the sternocleidomastoid muscle. The trajectory is parallel to the substance of the muscle along its undersurface. Apply gentle suction on the syringe until a rush of venous blood returns. Now repeat the procedure along the course of the seeker needle with the 2.5-inch, 18-gauge introducer needle on a 5-mL non-Luer-Lok syringe. Once venous puncture has been achieved, apply the Seldinger catheter-over-guidewire technique to pass the catheter, as described for subclavian venous catheterization.

8. Attach the IV fluid with Luer-Lok extension tubing, flush the line, and secure with sutures. Apply a sterile transparent adhesive dressing, and remove the rolled towel.

Femoral Venous Catheterization

1. Obtain written informed consent, if possible.

2. Position the patient supine and prepare the selected groin with iodophor solution.

3. Wash, gown, glove, and isolate the operative field with sterile towels.

4. The femoral vein is located medial to the common femoral artery just caudad to the inguinal ligament. The femoral arterial pulse serves as the landmark by which to locate the femoral vein. Palpate the femoral arterial pulse below the inguinal ligament with the index and middle fingers of the nondominant hand. Infil-

trate 1% lidocaine local anesthetic into the skin and subcutaneous tissues overlying the femoral vein. Pass the introducer needle into the vein and apply the Seldinger catheter-over-guidewire technique to introduce the catheter into the vein.

5. Attach IV fluid with sterile Luer-Lok extension tubing, flush the line, and secure with sutures. Apply a sterile transparent adhesive dressing.

FOLLOW-UP

1. Inspect the entry site daily for evidence of infection.

2. Change the dressing every 2 to 3 days.

3. With internal jugular or subclavian vein catheterization, a postprocedure portable anteroposterior chest roentgenogram is mandatory. It is important not only to order the film, but also to view it, to assess the position of the catheter and look for complications, such as pneumothorax and hemothorax.

4. With femoral vein catheterization, inspect the insertion site daily for evidence of hematoma.

5. Femoral vein catheters should be removed within 48 hours, if possible.

COMPLICATIONS

The overall rate of complications for central venous catheterization is approximately 10%; this rate is fairly consistent around the country, and includes both a major complication rate of 1% to 5%, and a minor complication rate of 5% to 9%. It is important to remember that while the rate is quite low, a finite mortality associated with this procedure exists.

1. *Infection.* Central venous catheter–related
   infection occurs with a frequency of 3% to 8%.

Factors associated with an increased frequency of infection include the following:

a. The length of time the catheter remains in place.

b. Use of the catheter for measurements of central venous pressure.

c. Use of the catheter for withdrawal of blood samples.

d. The technique of handling the catheter, its dressing, and its connections.

   Rigid adherence to aseptic techniques for catheter insertion and use, dressing changes, and regular replacement of intravenous fluids and tubing will minimize the risk of catheter-related infections. Application of antibiotic ointment at the catheter insertion site has been shown to increase the frequency of opportunistic, catheter-related infections, and such ointment should not be used. The use of a silver-impregnated collagen matrix cuff* at the catheter insertion site to prevent infection has limited application. These cuffs are useful for central venous catheters intended for long-term use, such as long-term intravenous antibiotic administration or hyperalimentation.

2. *Pneumothorax.* The frequency of pneumothorax as a complication of subclavian venous catheterization should be less than 2%. Technical expertise and a thorough knowledge of the relevant anatomy will minimize the incidence of pneumothorax. A small pneumothorax usually does not require intervention provided the patient is not on positive airway pressure and can be safely observed in an inpatient setting. A pneumothorax greater than 20% requires tube thoracostomy.

---

*Vita Cuff, Vitaphore Corp., San Carlos, CA.

3. *Hemothorax.* Bleeding into the pleural space can occur as the result of the following:

   a. Injury to the dome of the pleura in a patient with a coagulopathy or an abnormality in platelet number or function.

   b. Puncture of the subclavian vein or artery into the pleural space.

   c. A malpositioned catheter traversing the subclavian vein into the pleural space.

      Careful attention to the contraindications to the procedure, and technical expertise will minimize the risk. Management includes tube thoracostomy to evacuate the hemothorax, as well as attention to any existing coagulopathy.

4. *Chylothorax.* Injury to the lymphatic channels at the base of the neck can result in chylothorax. Lymphatic channel damage is infrequent but more likely to occur from left subclavian venipuncture. While chylothorax in this setting is usually self-limited and can be managed without intervention, the catheter should be removed.

5. *Intrapleural infusion of intravenous fluids.* This complication is related to malposition of the catheter within the pleural space and requires removal of the catheter.

6. *Cardiac dysrhythmias.* Passage of the guidewire into the heart can irritate the endocardium and induce abnormalities in cardiac rhythm. Attention to the length of guidewire inserted may prevent dysrhythmias. When an abnormal rhythm is recognized, pull the guidewire back into the superior vena cava. Be prepared to treat serious dysrhythmias with appropriate antiarrhythmic medications.

7. *Catheter malposition.* A catheter that follows an aberrant course should be repositioned or removed.

8. *Thrombosis.* Thrombosis of the subclavian vein requires removal of the catheter and anticoagulation, as clinically indicated.

Thrombosis of the catheter can be managed by gently flushing the catheter or by instilling a thrombolytic agent. If these measures are unsuccessful, remove the catheter. Iliofemoral venous thrombosis is a potentially morbid complication of femoral vein catheterization that may lead to pulmonary embolus and to chronic venous insufficiency of the lower extremity.

9. *Air embolism.* Sucking of air through the catheter or through the intravenous setup can be a catastrophic complication. Strict adherence to established techniques will prevent this complication. Should air embolization occur, position the patient in the left lateral decubitus position with Trendelenburg to prevent the air from moving into and occluding the right ventricular outflow tract.

10. *Pericardial tamponade.* Reports of central venous catheters eroding through the vessel wall exist. If the tip of the catheter is within the intrapericardial segment of the superior vena cava or in the right atrium or ventricle, a vascular erosion can result in bleeding or the instillation of intravenous fluid into the pericardium. The subsequent risk is pericardial tamponade. Careful attention to the position of the catheter will prevent this problem.

11. *Neurologic injury.* The brachial plexus is at risk during subclavian and internal jugular venipuncture. Technical expertise will prevent this complications. A brachial plexopathy is more likely to result from the pressure of an associated hematoma, rather than from direct injury. Nevertheless, the neurologic deficit can be permanent. The phrenic, vagus, and recurrent laryngeal nerves are at risk during internal jugular venipuncture. Careful attention to technique will minimize the risk of nerve injury.

12. *Arteriovenous fistula.* Simultaneous venous and arterial puncture, particularly in the neck, can

result in an arteriovenous fistula. When suspected, operative neck exploration and repair of the injury are required.

13. *Catheter embolization.* The risk of catheter embolization can be minimized by the use of the Seldinger catheter-over-guidewire technique.

14. *Hematoma.* Hematoma formation around the site of a femoral venous catheter can generally be managed with pressure to the site. On rare occasions, catheter removal might be required. Bleeding into the retroperitoneal space is, however, possible; this would result in substantial blood loss before becoming clinically apparent.

DOCUMENTATION

After the procedure, enter a note in the medical record documenting

a. The indications for the procedure.
b. The site of insertion.
c. The specific type of catheter used.
d. Any complications that occurred.
e. Interpretation of the postprocedure chest roentgenogram.

SUGGESTED READING

Bernard RW et al: Subclavian vein catheterization: a prospective study, I: non-infectious complications, *Ann Surg* 173:184, 1971.

Bernard RW et al: Subclavian vein catheterization: a prospective study, II: infectious complications, *Ann Surg* 173:191, 1971.

Bozzetti F: Central venous catheter sepsis, *Surg Gynecol Obstet* 161:293, 1985.

Ellis LM et al: Central venous catheter erosions, *Ann Surg* 209:475, 1989.

Feliciano DV et al: Major complications of percutaneous subclavian vein catheters, *Am J Surg* 138:869, 1979.

Getzen LC et al: Short term femoral vein catheterization: a safe alternative venous access? *Am J Surg* 138:875, 1979.

Kalso E: A short history of central venous catheterization, *Acta Anaesthesiol Scand [Suppl]* 81:7, 1985.

Linos DA et al: Subclavian vein: a golden route, *Mayo Clin Proc* 55:315, 1980.

Williams JF et al: Use of femoral venous catheters in critically ill adults; a prospective study, *Crit Care Med* 19:550, 1991.

3

Pulmonary Artery Catheterization

Debra L. Isaac, B.N., M.D.
Daniel J. Fintel, M.D.

INTRODUCTION

Evaluation of a patient's hemodynamic status plays an essential role in the critical care unit, both for patient assessment and for determination of appropriate therapeutic interventions. Hemodynamic monitoring includes both invasive and noninvasive methods of evaluating cardiovascular performance. Close observation of the patient by the clinician remains the most essential part of the hemodynamic assessment. Clinical assessments, however, may be relatively slow indicators of a change in hemodynamic status, and the use of pulmonary artery pressure monitoring is indicated when rapid, ongoing quantitative evaluation of the patient's hemodynamic status is required.

The flow-directed, balloon-tipped pulmonary artery catheter allows for assessment of intracardiac pressures at the bedside. The pulmonary artery (PA) catheter has multiple lumina for measurement, during insertion, of

1. Central venous pressure.
2. Right atrial pressure (RAP).

3. Right ventricular pressure.
4. Pulmonary artery pressure (PAP).

When properly situated, the PA catheter enables

a. Continuous monitoring of RAP and PAP.
b. Intermittent measurement of pulmonary artery occluded pressure for estimation of left ventricular end diastolic pressure. Because pressures measured at the right side of the heart are not always reliable determinants of left ventricular function, indirect measurement of left ventricular end diastolic pressure allows more accurate assessment of the critically ill patient.
c. Intermittent measurement of cardiac output by thermodilution technique.
d. Sampling of intracardiac blood.
e. The option of continuous measurement of mixed venous oxygen saturation (available with appropriate specialized PA catheters).
f. Placement of a temporary right ventricular pacing electrode.

Pulmonary artery catheterization is a simple bedside technique that does not require fluoroscopy in the majority of cases, because the balloon flotation device allows the catheter to be directed by blood flow from the right atrium into the right ventricle and subsequently into the PA. Continuous monitoring of the pressure at the distal tip of the PA catheter produces distinctive wave forms in each cardiac chamber that inform the clinician as to the position of the PA catheter within the heart and PA during insertion.

OBJECTIVE

Placement of a flow-directed, balloon-tipped, multi-lumen catheter by way of a central vein through the right side of the heart into the pulmonary artery.

Indications

1. Evaluation and management of acute heart failure.
2. Differentiation of ruptured ventricular septum from mitral regurgitation.
3. Evaluation of cardiac tamponade.
4. Intravascular fluid therapy in complex situations, such as the following.
   a. Burn injury.
   b. Severe hypovolemia.
   c. Hemorrhagic pancreatitis.
   d. Acute renal failure.
   e. Adult respiratory distress syndrome.
   f. Gram-negative sepsis.
   g. Extensive abdominal surgery with major fluid shifts.
   h. Right ventricular myocardial infarction.
5. Management of high-risk surgical patients with
   a. Pre-existing severe cardiac or pulmonary disease.
   b. Multiple trauma.
6. Management of high-risk surgical patients undergoing the following.
   a. Cardiac surgery.
   b. Vascular surgery.
   c. Prolonged or extensive surgical procedures.
7. Management of high-risk obstetric patients with the following conditions.
   a. Cardiac disease.
   b. Severe pregnancy-induced hypertension.
   c. Suspected abruptio placenta.

Contraindications

Although there are no absolute contraindications to the use of PA catheters, the potential benefit of catheter use must be weighed against the possible complications. Caution must be used in placing a PA catheter in patients with

   a. Recurrent septicemia.
   b. Immune deficiency.

c. Right-to-left intracardiac shunting.

d. Hypercoaguable states.

e. Left bundle branch block. Catheterization of the PA is associated with an increased risk of the development of complete heart block.

f. A history of tachyarrhythmias or ventricular arrhythmia, as insertion of a PA catheter may cause recurrence of these arrhythmias.

Emergency resuscitation equipment must, therefore, be nearby whenever a PA catheter is being inserted in any patient.

PREPARATION

Insertion

The insertion of a PA catheter requires central venous access (see Chapter 2). The PA catheter can also be placed by way of a peripheral venous cut-down technique. The usual sites for central venous access for the placement of a PA catheter include the internal jugular vein, subclavian vein, brachial vein (cut-down technique), or femoral vein. In general, the placement of a PA catheter at the bedside is most easily accomplished by way of the right internal jugular route, as this provides the most direct access to the right atrium and allows the clinician to take advantage of the curve of the PA catheter, which facilitates movement of the catheter from the right ventricle into the PA. Insertion of a PA catheter through a femoral venous site will most commonly require fluoroscopic guidance, as the catheter will require manual manipulation to pass from the inferior vena cave into the right atrium and ventricle and then into the PA.

Equipment

Assuming previous placement of a sheath introducer into the central venous system, the following equipment is required:

1. Sterile gowns, gloves, and mask.
2. Disinfecting solution and sterile drapes.
3. Pulmonary artery catheter (Fig 3–1).
4. Syringes, 3 mL and 10 mL.
5. Protective sterile sheath for the PA catheter.
6. Three three-way stopcocks.
7. Fluid-filled, low-compliance, pressure monitoring lines connected by way of an automatic flushing device to a pressurized bag filled with heparinized 0.9N saline.

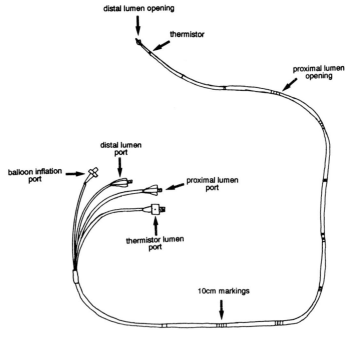

FIG 3–1.
Schematic illustrations of thermodilution-equipped Swan-Ganz type pulmonary artery catheter. (Used with permission of American Edwards Laboratories, Irvine, California.)

8. Pressure transducer connected to a pressure monitoring module capable of displaying real-time pressure wave forms and ordinal pressure valves.

9. Emergency resuscitation equipment, including anti-arrhythmic medications and cardioverter-defibrillator, must be within ready access.

Required Monitoring

The patient must be in a critical care unit setting, allowing

1. Continuous electrocardographic (EKG) monitoring.

2. Continuous venous pressure monitoring for the distal port of the PA catheter.

3. Continuous arterial blood pressure monitoring (desirable but not essential).

Required Laboratory Data

Laboratory data required prior to placement of central venous access line (see Chapter 2) must be obtained.

PROCEDURE

1. Explain the procedure to the patient and obtain consent.

2. Assemble and fill the monitoring lines that connect the transducer to the PA catheter (Fig 3–2). It is important that there are no air bubbles or leaks in this system; as their presence invalidates pressure readings.

3. Zero-balance and calibrate the transducer prior to insertion of the catheter.

4. Wash your hands and don sterile gown, gloves, and mask.

5. Clean the area around the central venous access site with iodophor solution and cover with sterile

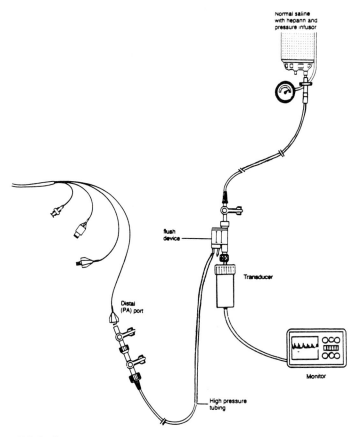

FIG 3-2.
A transducer and flush system set-up for pulmonary artery pressure monitoring.

drapes. The sterile drapes should cover the upper chest, neck, and face of the patient.

6. Prior to insertion, test the patency and integrity of the balloon on the PA catheter by inserting a 3-mL syringe into the balloon inflation port and injecting 1 cc of air. The balloon should inflate and remain inflated until the syringe is removed. Further confirmation of the integrity of the balloon can be achieved by placing the tip of the PA catheter, with the balloon still inflated, into a container of sterile normal saline. If there

is a leak in the balloon, small air bubbles may be seen escaping into the fluid. The syringe should then be removed from the balloon inflation port to allow the balloon to spontaneously deflate. It is important never to pull back on the syringe once it is in the inflation port, as deflating the balloon in this manner may cause trauma to and dysfunction of the balloon. The syringe should then be filled with 1 to 1.5 mL of air and replaced in the balloon inflation port, although the balloon should not be reinflated at this time.

7. Wipe the catheter with sterile gauze that has been wetted with heparinized saline. Prior to insertion of the PA catheter into the venous access introducer, place a protective sheath over the catheter. This sheath maintains sterility of the catheter and allows subsequent repositioning.

8. Hand the proximal portion of the PA catheter with the multiple ports to an unsterile assistant, while keeping the remaining part of the PA catheter sterile. The assistant then connects the pressure monitoring lines to both the distal and proximal PA ports, and fills them with the flush solution. If the PA catheter being used has additional ports (such as additional venous infusion ports), manually flush these with heparinized saline and close them off using stopcocks.

9. It is prudent at this time to make sure that the transducer and monitor are functioning properly by gently tapping the distal end of the PA catheter and looking for artifact on the monitor screen.

10. Insert the tip of the PA catheter into the previously placed introducer sheath. Once the tip of the catheter is in the vein, note the pressure tracing and ascertain the venous pressure. Pulmonary artery catheters are designed with a gentle curve that can be used to advantage during insertion. The curve should remain directed to allow easy flotation of the PA catheter from the right ventricle into the PA. For example, if the insertion is occurring by way of a right internal jugular line, the catheter should be inserted with the curve pointing to the left. Ideally, catheter advancement into

the PA should be as rapid as possible, as loss of catheter stiffness and curvature can occur with prolonged manipulation.

11. Advance the catheter approximately 15 cm if the insertion is through the internal jugular vein or subclavian vein, or approximately 40 cm if the insertion is through the antecubital fossa or femoral vein. At this time, the tip of the catheter is in the vicinity of the right atrium. Obtain a pressure tracing and note the actual pressure. Advance the catheter tip into the right atrium while observing the pressure tracing. The right atrial tracing is a low-pressure, low-excursion waveform in which distinct A and V waves should be visible. (Fig 3–3).

12. Inflate the balloon with 1 to 1.5 mL air and advance the catheter across the tricuspid valve into the right ventricle. Carefully monitor the EKG tracing, as entry of the PA catheter into the right ventricle may be associated with ventricular ectopy. As the catheter enters the right ventricle the pressure tracing will show a marked increase in pressure excursion. The systolic pressure is markedly increased, with the diastolic pressure remaining similar to the right atrial pressure, the

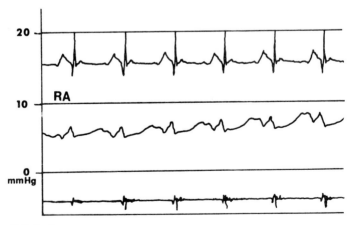

FIG 3–3.
Electrocardiogram and pressure tracing demonstrate waveform seen when the PA catheter tip is in the atrium *(RA)*.

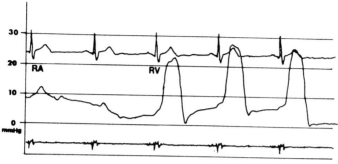

FIG 3–4.
Electrocardiogram and pressure tracing demonstrate waveform seen when the PA tip advances from right atrium *(RA)* into the right ventricle *(RV)*.

result being a markedly biphasic wave form as shown in Fig 3–4. Pause briefly to measure right ventricular pressures; avoid prolonged presence of the PA catheter tip in the right ventricular cavity, as this may be arrhythmogenic.

13. Continue advancement of the PA catheter into the PA demonstrated by a change in waveform showing an increase in the diastolic pressure with resulting diminution in the excursion of the waveform. The PA systolic pressure remains essentially the same as the right ventricular systolic pressure (Fig 3–5). After a

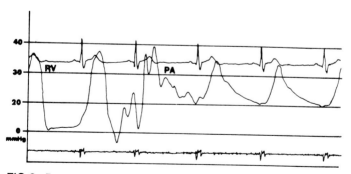

FIG 3–5.
Electrocardiogram and pressure tracing demonstrate waveform seen when the PA tip advances from right ventricle *(RV)* to pulmonary artery *(PA)*.

brief pause to note and record PA pressures and waveform, slowly advance the catheter, with the balloon remaining inflated, until the PA waveform changes to a
low-amplitude wave associated with occlusion of the
PA (Fig 3–6). At this time, if insertion is through the internal jugular or subclavian vein, the PA catheter will
have been inserted between 40 to 55 cm in most patients. Ten-centimeter markings are present on the PA
catheter to allow assessment of length of catheter advancement. Do not advance the PA catheter farther
once the pulmonary artery occluded pressure (PAOP)
tracing has been obtained. Inadvertent further advancement of the PA catheter will result in "over wedging" of the catheter with resultant flattening of the
PAOP wave form and steadily increasing pressure (Fig
3–7). If this occurs, deflate the balloon and pull back
the PA catheter several centimeters, reinflate the balloon, and advance to a PAOP position again. Once an
acceptable PAOP tracing has been obtained, deflate the
balloon, and the pressure tracing should spontaneously
return to the biphasic PA pressure form. Subsequent
slow inflation of the balloon with not more than 1.5 cc
of air should result in reappearance of the PAOP tracing. Note the PAOP pressure.

14. Attach the proximal end of the protective sheath
over the PA catheter to the introducer sheath.

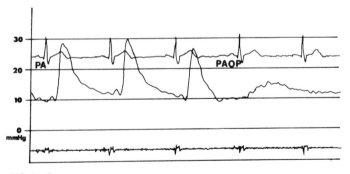

FIG 3–6.
Electrocardiogram and pressure tracing demonstrate waveform seen
when PA catheter tip advances from pulmonary artery *(PA)* to pulmonary
artery occluded pressure *(PAOP)* position.

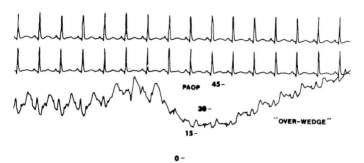

FIG 3–7.
Electrocardiogram and pressure tracing demonstrate pulmonary artery waveform followed by PAOP and "over wedging" of the PA catheter.

15. Note the distance the PA catheter has been introduced. Coil the external remaining part of the PA catheter and securely fasten with a sterile dressing to prevent accidental dislodgement.

Potential Problems During PA Catheter Placement

1. *Failure to enter the right ventricle.* If the PA catheter has been advanced more than the expected length to enter the right ventricle without resultant change of the pressure tracing to indicate RV pressures, it is possible that the PA catheter has entered the inferior vena cava. Deflate the balloon and pull the PA catheter back to approximately 10 or 15 cm, assuming internal jugular or subclavian insertion. Reinflate the balloon and readvance the PA catheter. If the same problem should reoccur, again deflate the balloon and remove the PA catheter entirely. Check that the direction of the curve of the PA catheter allows the catheter to naturally curve up from the right atrium into the right ventricle and the PA.

In patients with marked tricuspid regurgitation, there may be significant difficulty in advancing the catheter across the tricuspid valve, and fluoroscopic guidance may be required.

2. *Failure to advance the PA catheter from the right ventricle into the PA.* If the PA catheter has been ad-

vanced more than 40 to 45 cm (assuming internal jugular or subclavian insertion sites) and the PA tracing has
not been achieved, deflate the balloon and pull the PA
catheter back to the right atrium. Reinflate the balloon
and attempt readvancement as described earlier. **The
balloon must be deflated before the PA is pulled back
because of the danger of injury to valve leaflets with
the inflated balloon.** In patients with a dilated right
ventricle, the PA catheter may tend to curl in the right
ventricle rather than advancing into the PA. On occa-
sion, difficulty in passing the PA catheter from the right
ventricle into the PA can be overcome by placing the
patient on his/her left side, or asking the patient to take
a deep breath. Repeated difficulty in advancing the PA
catheter warrants fluoroscopic guidance.

3. *Failure to obtain a PAOP tracing once in the PA.*
Occasionally, a PAOP tracing cannot be obtained, particularly in patients with primary pulmonary hypertension. In patients with significant mitral regurgitation,
where the presence of a large V-wave in the PAOP tracing may mimic the PA pressure tracing (Fig 3–8), a distinct change in the pressure wave form from PA to
PAOP may not be appreciated.

4. *Respiratory fluctuation in pressure tracing baseline.*

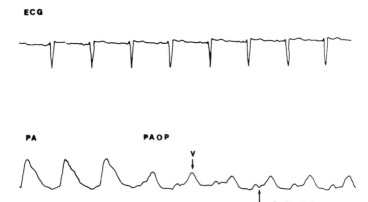

FIG 3–8.
Tracing of *PA* and *PAOP* waveform in a patient with mitral regurgitation.
Note prominent "V" wave.

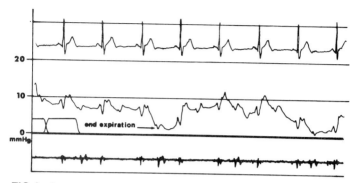

FIG 3–9.
Electrocardiogram and pressure tracing demonstrate PAOP waveform with marked respiratory variation. Measurement of PAOP should be taken at end expiration, as indicated on the tracing.

In some patients, particularly those with respiratory distress, a marked fluctuation of the PA tracing may be seen during the phases of respiration. This "respiratory variation," an artifact that occurs because the transducer is referenced to atmospheric pressure rather than airway pressure, results in measurement errors that do not reflect true hemodynamic variations. This measurement error can be reduced by selecting and measuring portions of the waveform that occur when airway pressure is relatively low and stable, as occurs at end expiration. Although some monitoring systems are equipped with computer algorithms, that attempt to compensate for respiratory variation, it is usually best to select end expiratory waveforms and measure the pressures manually (Fig 3–9.)

FOLLOW-UP

1. After placement of the PA catheter, obtain a chest roentgenogram to document proper positioning of the tip of the catheter. The PA catheter should be seen proceeding from the access site through the right atrium and right ventricle into the PA. The tip of the PA catheter should be within the main trunk of either the left or right PA and should not extend into more peripheral branches.

2. Continuous display of the PA pressure tracing and frequent examination of the PA catheter position at the insertion site are necessary to ensure that the PA catheter has not been inadvertently advanced or pulled back. Any repositioning of the PA catheter must be done with strict aseptic precautions. If the monitor shows a PAOP tracing, check the PA catheter to ensure that the balloon has not been inadvertently inflated and that the catheter flush system remains functional. If the balloon is not inflated, gradually pull back the PA catheter until the PA waveform is observed again. The PA catheter may also migrate back into the right ventricle, which may result in ventricular arrhythmias. If this should occur, immediately inflate the balloon and readvance the catheter into the PA. If the PA cannot be reentered immediately, deflate the balloon and pull back the catheter to the right atrium before attempting repositioning.

3. Continuous monitoring of PA pressure can be maintained for up to 3 days, at which time, if hemodynamic monitoring is still indicated, replace the PA catheter to decrease risk of infection or thrombosis. Maintenance of a PA catheter within the heart and PA is not without risk of complications; therefore, it is prudent to remove the PA catheter as soon as the patient's condition allows discontinuation of invasive hemodynamic monitoring.

4. Obtain a chest roentgenogram daily to evaluate the position of the tip of the PA catheter.

5. Inspect the catheter insertion site daily for evidence of infection. If the site appears infected, remove the catheter and introducer sheath to a different clean site. Send the tip of the catheter and introducer sheath for microbiologic studies.

COMPLICATIONS

1. Complications associated with obtaining central venous access (see Chapter 2).

2. Potential complications of hemodynamic monitoring with PA catheters, related to both insertion and maintenance of the catheter. These are relatively infrequent, and for the most part, of minor significance (Table 3–1). They include the following.

   a. Ventricular arrhythmias, transient right bundle branch block, or complete heart block, which may not respond to the removal of the PA catheter.

   b. Valvular damage, which can occur during insertion of a PA catheter, particularly if repeated attempts at advancement are made or if the PA catheter is inadvertently pulled back with the balloon still inflated.

   c. In very rare instances, knotting of the PA catheter within the right atrium or right ventricle secondary to looping of the catheter within the heart. If this is suspected, usually on the basis of inability to withdraw the PA catheter or advance into the PA, fluoroscopic guidance is required for further manipulation of the PA catheter. This adjustment should be attempted only by persons with experience.

TABLE 3–1.

Potential Complications of Hemodynamic Monitoring With a Pulmonary Artery Catheter

Arrhythmias
Ventricular arrhythmias
Transient right bundle branch block
Complete heart block
Valvular damage
Knotting of the catheter
Perforation of atrial or ventricular wall
Pulmonary air embolus
Pulmonary thromboembolus
Pulmonary artery injury
Pulmonary infarction
Catheter-related sepsis

Rarely, a local surgical procedure may be required for removal of the PA catheter.

d. Perforation of the atrial or ventricular wall is a potential but very rare complication.

e. Pulmonary air embolus associated with improper flushing of the PA catheter prior to insertion, or attempted inflation of a ruptured balloon.

f. Pulmonary thromboembolism can occur if a thrombus formed on the PA catheter should dislodge. Catheter thrombus formation may be more common in patients who are hypercoagulable or in whom the PA catheter has been in place for a prolonged period of time.

g. Catheter-related sepsis can occur both as a result of the disruption of the skin at the insertion site, with subsequent tracking into the circulation, and by thrombus formation along the course of the PA catheter, serving as a nidus for infection.

h. Injury to the PA, probably related to overinflation of the balloon or over-advancement of the PA catheter, can occur during catheter insertion or maintenance. Rupture of the PA usually presents as sudden, unexpected hemoptysis, which may be massive and result in life-threatening hemodynamic instability. If PA rupture is suspected, supportive measures—including fluid and blood product administration and airway protection—must be instituted. Emergency pulmonary angiography and further management, including surgery, may be required in the case of significant PA injury.

i. Pulmonary infarction may also occur, particularly if the catheter is maintained in the PAOP position for a prolonged period of time.

DOCUMENTATION

Write a procedure note in the patient's chart which includes the following:

1. Indication for PA catheterization.
2. Choice of site of venous access.
3. Size and type of PA catheter inserted.
4. Distance the PA catheter was advanced to achieve the PAOP position.
5. Any complications or difficulties encountered during catheter placement.

Record and attach the initial intracardiac pressure tracings and values to the patient's medical record. Document subsequent pressure values and additional hemodynamic values (cardiac output and derived cardiac calculations) on a flow sheet, which allows ongoing assessment of patient's status and response to therapeutic interventions.

SUGGESTED READING

Amin DK et al: The Swan-Ganz catheter: indications for insertion, *J Crit Illness* 1:54, 1986.

Bustin DL: *Hemodynamic monitoring for critical care*, Norwalk, Conn, 1986, Appleton Century Crofts.

Forrester JS et al: Medical therapy of acute myocardial infarction by application of hemodynamic subsets, part 1, *N Engl J Med* 295:1356, 1976.

Forrester JS et al: Medical therapy of acute myocardial infarction by application of hemodynamic subsets, part 2, *N Engl J Med* 295:1404, 1976.

Friesinger GC et al: Clinical competence in hemodynamic monitoring: a statement for physicians from the ACP/ACC/AHA Task Force on clinical privileges in cardiology, *J Am Coll Cardiol* 15:1460, 1990.

Iberti TJ et al: A prospective study on the use of the pulmonary artery catheter in a medical intensive care unit, its effect on diagnosis and therapy, *Crit Care Med* 11:238, 1983.

Matthay MA et al: Bedside catheterization of the pulmonary artery: risks compared with benefits, *Ann Intern Med* 109:826, 1988.

Nadeau S, Noble WH: Misinterpretation of pressure measurements from the pulmonary artery catheter, *J Can Anesthesiol* 33:352, 1986.

Puri VK et al: Complications of vascular catheterization in the critically ill, *Crit Care Med* 8:495, 1980.

Shah KB et al: A review of pulmonary artery catheterization in 6245 patients, *Anesthesiology* 61:271, 1984.

Vender JS: Invasive cardiac monitoring, *Crit Care Clin* 4:455, 1988.

4

Thoracentesis

Michael H. Albrink, M.D.

INTRODUCTION

Thoracentesis is an essential part of the diagnostic and therapeutic acumen of the critical care physician. Aspiration of pleural fluid is often the only way a diagnosis can be made. Pulmonary volume loss by extrinsic compression from effusions can be a severely limiting factor and add to respiratory insufficiency.

OBJECTIVE

To place and secure a catheter in the pleural space to sample (diagnostic) or drain (therapeutic) pleural effusions.

Indications

Thoracentesis is indicated in

1. Pleural effusions of unclear cause.
2. Large or symptomatic pleural effusions that do not respond to typical measures of fluid restriction and diuretics.
3. Pleural effusions in patients with unexplained fever.

Contraindications

1. Local chest wall infection with cellulitis.
2. Relative contraindications include the following.
   a. Coagulopathy.
   b. Previous chest surgery with pleural adhesions.

Thoracentesis is associated with greater risk in patients on positive pressure ventilation.

PREPARATION

Careful physical examination of the patient is mandatory, with particular attention to the chest examination. Locating the effusion can be achieved with the following:

1. Percussion of the thoracic spaces in a multitude of positions is needed to determine the location of the effusions and to determine if loculation is present.
2. Chest roentgenograms in the upright, lateral decubitus, and true lateral projections are needed to show the true location of the fluid collections.
3. Ultrasonography may be quite helpful in patients who are unable to be placed in the various roentgenographic positions. Ultrasound guidance can also help in needle placement during performance of the procedure.

Equipment

1. Sterile gloves.
2. Drapes.
3. Iodophor solution.
4. Local anesthetic.
5. Syringes.
6. Needles.
7. Specimen containers (generally needed).

There are many excellent, commercially prepared trays that are reasonably comprehensive. Most physicians recommend a modified Seldinger technique with a guidewire because, in theory, it offers a lower risk of pneumothorax.

Required Monitoring

Each clinical situation will require some form of monitoring, ranging from simple observation to sophisticated computerized multimodality screens. No specific monitoring is needed for thoracentesis. It may be performed in the patient's room, in the emergency department, or in the intensive care unit. Additional monitoring other than the presence of the physician and help from nursing colleagues is not necessary.

Required Laboratory Data

1. Blood studies, such as prothrombin time, partial thromboplastin time, and platelet count should be ordered.

2. At least two views of chest roentgenograms are needed.

3. A normal bleeding time may supplant the need for coagulation studies.

4. Evaluation of several serum parameters may aid in the laboratory evaluation of pleural fluid. These include serum lactic dehydrogenase (LDH), protein, glucose, and amylase measurements.

PROCEDURE

1. Introduce yourself to the patient and carefully describe the procedure, including risks, benefits, and possible complications.

2. If possible, position the patient comfortably in a sitting position with his/her arms resting on a bedside tray stand. If the patient's medical condition prohibits this position, place the patient in a position that ex-

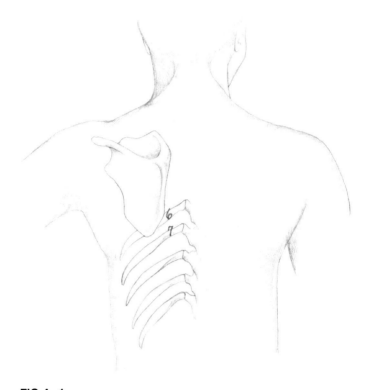

FIG 4–1.
Site for thoracocentesis at the sixth to seventh intercostal space posteriorly, inferior to the scapula.

poses the area to be punctured, with the effusion in a relatively dependent position.

3. Choose the area for aspiration by a combination of clinical factors and radiographic views (roentgenography, ultrasonography). With the patient sitting, this area is typically the sixth to seventh interspace or just inferior to the tip of the scapula (Fig 4–1). Don sterile gloves. Cleanse widely around the thoracentesis site with iodophor solution. Apply sterile drapes around the site so that they will not fall from the sitting patient.

4. Anesthetize the precise area of aspiration with 1% lidocaine, progressing from superficial (Fig 4–2) to

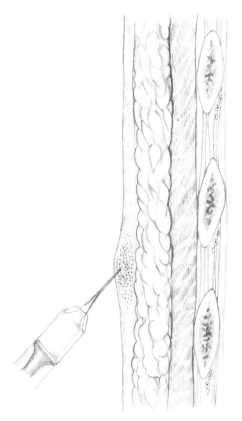

FIG 4–2.
Raise a skin weal with local anesthesia at the site for thoracocentesis.

deeper layers of the chest wall (Fig 4–3). Aspirate the needle, inject anesthetic solution, and advance the needle. The pleura is particularly sensitive and is also difficult to anesthetize.

5. Enter the pleural cavity between the ribs. Stay as close to the superior border of the rib as possible to avoid inadvertent puncture of the intercostal vessels.

6. Once in the pleural space, you should be able to aspirate a free flow of fluid into the local anesthetic syringe. Carefully mark the exact depth of the needle

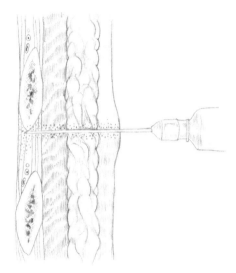

FIG 4–3.
Infiltrate the full thickness of the chest wall with local anesthesia.

within the chest wall at which pleural fluid first returns. This depth can be extrapolated to the insertion of later devices.

7. Attempt to instill additional local anesthetic solution into the parietal pleura; inject in a back-and-forth fashion. Large effusions will help protect the underlying lung from puncture.

8. Attach a syringe to a thin-walled needle and insert through the anesthetized area with continuous traction on the barrel of the syringe (Fig 4–4). You should have a rough approximation of the required depth from the mark on the needle used for administration of local anesthetic solution. Once free flow of pleural fluid into the syringe is obtained, insert a guidewire through the needle into the pleural space.

9. Remove the thin-walled needle and make a small skin incision with a scalpel directly at the guidewire entry site. Pass a dilator over the wire and dilate the tract. Remove the dilator and pass a thoracentesis catheter over the guidewire (Fig 4–5). Ideal thoracentesis

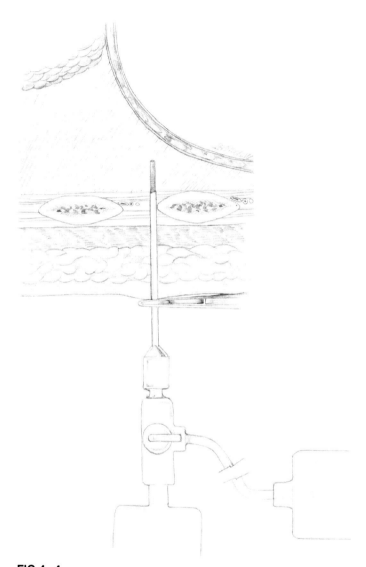

FIG 4–4.
Section through the chest wall and pleural space showing the thoracocentesis needle entering the pleural space with guide wire passed through needle.

FIG 4–5.
Section through the chest wall and pleural space showing introduction of
the catheter into the pleural space.

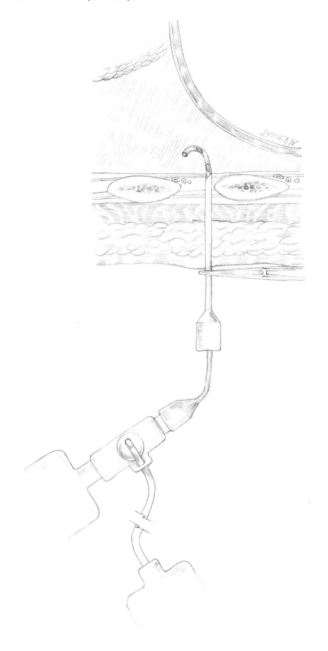

catheters have multiple sideholes and may have a curved or "pigtail" configuration.

10. To prevent air from entering the pleural cavity ensure that all the holes in the thoracentesis catheter are in the chest. Place a three-way stopcock on the proximal end of the catheter and close to the outside.

11. Prior to aspirating or removing large amounts of fluid, attach the catheter to the chest wall with skin sutures. After this is accomplished, large amounts of pleural fluid can be removed.

12. Attach sterile intravenous fluid administration tubing to the three-way stopcock and connect to either an empty sterile basin or a collecting bottle. The fluid can be aspirated manually with a syringe or allowed to drain passively by gravity.

13. Apply a sterile dressing over the puncture site and obtain a chest roentgenogram to document the amount of drainage and the presence or absence of a pneumothorax.

14. Send fluid specimens for Gram stain, culture and sensitivity, cell count with differential, LDH, protein, and specific gravity testing. Measurement of pH and amylase may be helpful in certain instances.

15. Remove the catheter once the desired therapeutic effect has been achieved or the appropriate diagnostic samples obtained. Cover the puncture site with a sterile dressing.

FOLLOW-UP

The catheter and the wound should be inspected on a daily basis, with a particular emphasis on rigid fixation of the catheter. Much of the follow-up activity is predicated on the actual results of fluid analysis. Infected collections must be drained and a source identified. Malignant effusions may be treated with sclerosis as a palliative measure, although this is not often effective. Pleural effusions are common on the left side of the chest in cases of severe pancreatitis, but no specific therapy is required. Pleural effusions with a pH lower than 7.20 generally indicate an infectious cause.

COMPLICATIONS

Common complications of thoracentesis include

1. Pneumothorax.
2. Hemothorax.
3. Intercostal vessel laceration.
4. Chest wall bleeding with hematoma formation.
5. Bronchopleural fistula (the most feared and difficult to treat).

DOCUMENTATION

Write a note in the Progress section of the patient's chart that includes

1. Indication for procedure.
2. Preparatory examination and investigations employed to identify the site of the effusion.
3. Site of chest wall puncture.
4. Amount and nature of local anesthetic solution administered.
5. Amount of fluid removed from the pleural space.
6. List of the tests ordered on the aspirated fluid.
7. Postprocedure chest roentgenographic findings.
8. Complications encountered, if any.

SUGGESTED READING

Brooks JW: Complications of pulmonary and chest wall resection. In Greenfield L, editor: *Complications in surgery and trauma*, Philadelphia, 1990, JB Lippincott.

Chakko SC et al: Treatment of congestive failure: its effect on pleural fluid chemistry, *Chest* 95:798, 1989.

Hood RM et al: *Thoracic trauma,* Philadelphia, 1989, WB Saunders.

Rasmussen OS et al: Ultrasound guided puncture of pleural fluid collections and superficial thoracic masses, *Eur J Radiol* 9:91, 1989.

5

Paracentesis and Diagnostic Peritoneal Lavage

Michael H. Albrink, M.D.

INTRODUCTION

Sampling of free fluid from the peritoneal cavity is a useful diagnostic technique. Paracentesis, either by needle or catheter aspiration of fluid, is used in the diagnosis of a variety of conditions including bacterial peritonitis, hemorrhage, portal hypertension, malignancy, and pancreatitis. Although needle paracentesis is effective, catheter placement is the more common technique. This discussion will focus on catheter paracentesis.

Diagnostic peritoneal lavage (DPL), introduced by Root in 1967, is a modification of catheter paracentesis involving infusion of saline into the peritoneal cavity. The technique is commonly used in the diagnosis of traumatic hemoperitoneum. The DPL procedure has been shown to have sensitivities and specificities of 95% to 99% in many studies.

OBJECTIVE

To safely place and secure a catheter in the peritoneal cavity for obtaining fluid for both diagnostic and therapeutic purposes. In addition to placing a catheter, diagnostic peritoneal lavage involves infusion of normal saline into the peritoneal cavity with return of appropriate amounts for diagnostic studies.

Indications

1. Paracentesis.
   a. Unexplained ascites.
   b. Ascites with unexplained fever.
   c. Unexplained hypotension.
   d. Pancreatitis with ascites.
   e. Suspected bacterial peritonitis.
   f. Myxedema ascites.
   g. Aspiration of peritoneal fluid in tense ascites resulting in respiratory compromise; this frequently brings symptomatic improvement.
2. Diagnostic peritoneal lavage.
   a. Unexplained hypotension and an unexplained drop in the hematocrit in injured patients.
   b. Equivocal physical examination of the abdomen in patients with pelvic fractures, lower rib fractures, and lumbar spine fractures, conditions which may significantly alter the physical examination of the abdomen.
   c. Patients in whom physical examination of the abdomen will be either inconvenient or impractical, such as lengthy general anesthesia for extra-abdominal operations, or radiologic procedures such as angiography or embolization.
   d. Patients in whom abdominal examination is frequently unreliable, for example, patients with spinal cord injuries, head injuries with altered state of consciousness, or intoxication.

Contraindications

1. Paracentesis.
   a. Significant intra-abdominal adhesions from previous surgery.
   b. Severe coagulopathy.
   c. Lack of clinical relevance (will not be acted upon regardless of results).
2. Diagnostic peritoneal lavage.
   a. Absolute contraindications.
      (1) Patient in whom abdominal exploration will be undertaken regardless of DPL results, such as obvious evisceration, gunshot wounds, marked peritonitis with injury.
      (2) Conditions for which no operation will be undertaken regardless of the results, such as brain death, terminal cancer, "do not resuscitate" status.
   b. Relative contraindications.
      (1) Pelvic fractures.
      (2) Advanced pregnancy.
      (3) Previous abdominal surgery with adhesions.
      (4) Morbid obesity.
      (5) Cirrhosis with documented coagulopathy.

PREPARATION

Careful physical examination of the abdomen is mandatory. This should include the presence or absence of surgical scars, caput medusae, fluid wave, shifting dullness, and organomegaly. Coagulation parameters should be noted and deficiencies corrected if possible. The urinary bladder should be emptied either by voluntary means or by one-time catheterization. Ultrasonic examination may be useful in diagnosis of ascites, as both physical examination and roentgenograms are often unreliable in ascites detection. Ultrasound may be quite useful in locating fluid collections and is of special utility where there are adhesions at sites of previous scar/surgical incisions.

Equipment

1. Sterile gloves.
2. Sterile towels and drapes.
3. Syringes with needles.
4. Local anesthetic (lidocaine, 1%).
5. "J-wire."
6. Collection tubes for samples.
7. Appropriate culture media.
8. Paracentesis catheter, or peritoneal dialysis catheter for DPL.
9. Iodophor solution.
10. Non-Luer-Lok syringes.
11. Additional equipment for DPL, including the following.
    a. Intravenous tubing without a one-way valve.
    b. Scalpel.
    c. Hemostats.
    d. Forceps.
    e. Suture material.
    f. One liter normal saline.

Comprehensive packages containing all necessary equipment exist and can be useful and convenient.

Required Monitoring

None.

Required Laboratory Data

Evaluation of prothrombin time, partial thrombo-plastin time, and platelet counts are desirable; however, emergency conditions may both preclude the tests and pre-empt the correction of deficiencies. Clinical judgment is necessary in these situations.

PROCEDURE

1. Introduce yourself to the patient and explain the procedure.
2. Place the patient in the supine position with the head slightly elevated for patient comfort.
3. Cleanse the abdomen with iodophor solution and drape in a sterile fashion.
4. Select the exact site for abdominal puncture with caution to avoid surgical scars, obvious caput medusae, and the anticipated locations of the inferior epigastric arteries. A site in the lower midline is preferable, but either lower quadrant is acceptable. The goal of placing a catheter into the pelvis is the objective.

    The site of DPL may be altered from infraumbilical to supraumbilical or paramedian if any of a number of conditions are present, including pregnancy, pelvic fractures, and previous surgery with scars.
5. Inject local anesthetic, raising a skin weal, followed by deeper instillation into the subcutaneous tissues.
6. Attach a non-Luer-Lok syringe to a thin-walled needle. Using a "Z-track" technique, insert the needle into the peritoneal cavity with continuous gentle aspiration on the syringe. Intraperitoneal position will be shown by free flow of peritoneal fluid.
7. Detach the thin-walled needle from the non-Luer-Lok syringe with caution to avoid moving the needle either in or out. Insert a soft J-tipped guidewire through the needle into the peritoneal cavity and slide the needle out over the guidewire.
8. Slide the paracentesis catheter over the guidewire using a twisting motion. It may be necessary to insert a dilator over the guidewire before inserting the paracentesis catheter
9. Connect a syringe to the catheter and aspirate as

much peritoneal fluid as is needed to complete the indicated studies (red blood cell count, white blood cell count, bilirubin, amylase and Gram stain).

10. Remove the catheter and apply an occlusive dressing. In some cases it may be necessary to place a "purse-string" suture around the puncture site to prevent persistent leakage of peritoneal fluid.

11. To perform DPL, initially follow steps 1 through 5 of the foregoing procedure. Thereafter proceed as follows.

    a. The DPL procedure is typically performed by the open technique in the lower midline position. Incisions closer to the umbilicus are advised, and will lessen the amount of properitoneal fat between the fascia and the peritoneum.

    b. Incise the skin in the midline. Continue the incision down to the fascia. Open the fascia for a distance of 2 to 3 cm.

    c. With blunt dissection, spread the properitoneal fat until the peritoneum is visualized. This maneuver is aided by use of two hemostats with blades spread at right angles to each other.

    d. The peritoneum will appear a dull grey color. Open the peritoneum just enough to allow passage of the catheter.

    e. The DPL procedure is usually performed with a temporary dialysis catheter. Pass the temporary peritoneal dialysis catheter through the peritoneal opening and direct the catheter in such a manner that the tip of the catheter "hugs" the anterior abdominal wall (Fig 5–1). After the catheter has been inserted 5 to 10 cm, rotate the catheter 180°, which will result in the catheter tip being directed into the pelvis (Fig 5–2). Avoid the use of rigid stylets in the peritoneal catheter, as the risk of

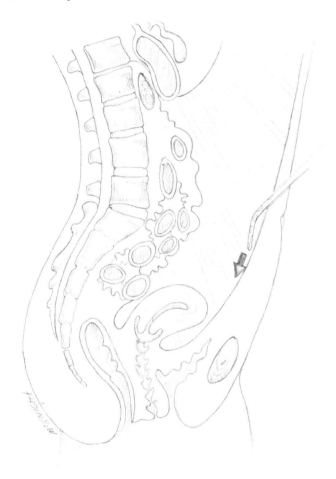

FIG 5–1.
Median section through the lower abdomen showing the catheter tip being introduced through the abdominal wall and directed so as to keep the tip against the abdominal wall.

perforation of a viscus is increased with their use.

f. Attach a connecting tube and syringe to the catheter and aspirate. Free flow of 10 mL of blood indicates a positive tap and suggests the need for operative intervention.

g. Connect an intravenous delivery set to the DPL

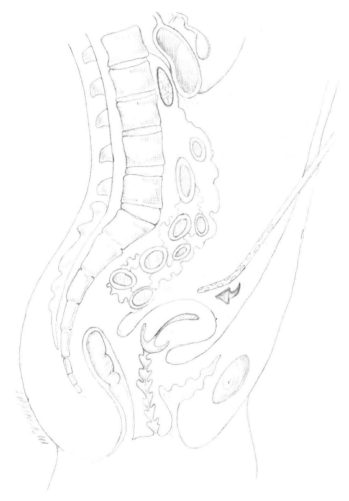

FIG 5–2.
Median section through the lower abdomen showing the catheter tip rotated 180°, thereby directed into the pelvis.

catheter and infuse 1 L or 10 mL/kg, whichever is the lesser amount, of 0.9% saline into the peritoneal cavity.

h. Just before the fluid is completely infused, lower the infusion bag to the floor without allowing air to enter the delivery tubing.

Lowering the infusion bag will let the lavage fluid efflux from the peritoneal cavity by a siphon effect. It is important to hold the catheter in place without movement. Movement of the catheter may allow the intestine to come between the catheter and the "pool" of lavage fluid. Remove as much fluid as possible; 250 mL is the minimum amount required for diagnostic accuracy.

i. Collect and send lavage effluent samples for red blood cell count, white blood cell count, bilirubin values, amylase values, and Gram stain.

j. If the lavage is negative for disease, close the fascia with 0-polypropylene sutures. Close the skin with sutures or staples. If the study is positive and a laparotomy is to be performed, it is not necessary to close the wound.

k. If temporary peritoneal dialysis or lavage is planned (acute renal failure, pancreatic ascites), leave the catheter in situ and close the wound with a water-tight seal.

FOLLOW-UP

Daily inspection of the puncture site and daily physical examination of the abdomen are mandatory. Clinical vigilance is needed to diagnose any complication.

COMPLICATIONS

1. Visceral perforation.
2. Enterocutaneous fistula.
3. Peritonitis.
4. Intra-abdominal abscess.
5. Intra-abdominal hemorrhage.
6. Abdominal wall hematoma.
7. Injury to inferior epigastric artery.
8. Urinary bladder injury.

DOCUMENTATION

Write a note in the chart that includes the following:

1. Indication for procedure.
2. Steps taken, i.e., paracentesis or DPL.
3. Site on abdominal wall and reason for choice of site.
4. Volume of fluid aspirated for paracentesis.
5. If DPL performed record volume of saline infused and volume returned.
6. Nature of fluid obtained.
7. Samples sent for laboratory testing.
8. Any complications that may have occurred.

SUGGESTED READING

Akriadis EA, Runyon BA: Utility of an algorithm in differentiating spontaneous from secondary bacterial peritonitis, *Gastroenterology* 98:127, 1990.

Alaniz C: Management of cirrhotic ascites, *Clin Pharmacol Ther* 8:645, 1989.

Hoefs JC: Diagnostic paracentesis: a potent clinical tool, *Gastroenterology* 98:230, 1990.

Neighbor ML: Ascites, *Emerg Med Clin North Am* 7:683, 1989.

Ross GJ et al: Sonographically guided paracentesis for palliation of symptomatic malignant ascites, *AJR* 153:1309, 1989.

6

Percutaneous Pericardiocentesis

Robert C. Hendel, M.D.

INTRODUCTION

Pericardiocentesis, the withdrawal of fluid from the pericardial space, has been performed for more than 150 years. While direct surgical approaches provide accurate means of pericardial fluid removal, these techniques require both time and specialized skills and entail significant risk of infectious complications. Percutaneous pericardiocentesis can be performed rapidly and with minimal equipment, but there is potential for significant complications with this "blind" approach, due to the uncertainty of locating the pericardial effusion without damaging vital structures. Modifications of the early technique have resulted in a method that is almost always successful and is infrequently associated with adverse effects. The surgical method is still favored, however, for the definitive treatment of purulent pericarditis and traumatic tamponade.

OBJECTIVE

Removal of pericardial fluid for diagnostic and/or therapeutic purposes.

Indications

1. Diagnostic.
   a. Suspicion of infectious process.
   b. Suspicion of neoplastic disease.
2. Therapeutic.
   a. Relief of pericardial tamponade.
   b. Treatment of malignant effusion.

Contraindications

In the setting of life-threatening cardiac tamponade, there are obviously no contraindications to pericardiocentesis. However, when performed for diagnostic purposes or in less urgent circumstances, the following are relative contraindications:

   a. Coagulopathy.
   b. Electrolyte imbalance (hypokalemia).
   c. Infection.

PREPARATION

Fluoroscopy is highly useful and is the preferred guidance technique by which to position an intrapericardial catheter. The ideal location for the performance of pericardiocentesis is a cardiac catheterization laboratory, where radiologic and hemodynamic monitoring facilities are optimal. Despite these recommendations, pericardiocentesis can be performed safely at the bedside or in the intensive care unit.

Equipment

1. Sterile sponges.
2. Providone-iodine solution.
3. Mask, sterile gown, and gloves.
4. Sterile towels and drapes.
5. Ten milliliters lidocaine, 1% solution.

6. Needles.
   a. 25-Gauge, 0.625 inch.
   b. 21-Gauge, 1.5 inch.
   c. 14- or 16-Gauge, 3-inch, short bevel.
7. Syringes.
   a. Ten milliliter.
   b. Fifty milliliter.
8. Three-way stopcock.
9. Guidewire, 0.038 J-tipped.
10. Dilator, 7 or 8 F.
11. Short pigtail catheter, 7 or 8 F.
12. One-way valve tubing connector.
13. Tubing connection to drainage bag.
14. One-liter drainage bag.
15. Pressure monitoring transducer with fluid-filled connecting tubing.
16. Number 11 scalpel blade.
17. Sterile alligator clip and cable.
18. Electrocardiographic (EKG) machine.
19. Specimen tubes, for the following.
    a. Hematocrit.
    b. Culture.
    c. Cytology.
    d. Chemistry.
20. Silk suture, 3-0.
21. Tape and antibiotic ointment.
22. Resuscitation equipment.
    a. Defibrillator.
    b. Intubation tray.
    c. Emergency drugs.
23. Sedative medications.

Required Monitoring

1. Continuous EKG monitoring.
2. Frequent blood pressure assessment.
3. Intra-arterial pressure monitoring (recommended).
4. A pulmonary artery catheter. This is desirable to document the hemodynamic consequences of cardiac

tamponade and the effects of pericardiocentesis. Furthermore, it enables close observation for potential complications such as hemopericardium.

Required Laboratory Data

In the setting of an emergency procedure, no laboratory information is required. Under elective circumstances, the following are desirable:

1. Coagulation profile consisting of prothrombin time, partial thromboplastin time, and platelet count.
2. Serum electrolytes, especially potassium.

PROCEDURE

1. Confirm presence and location of pericardial effusion by echocardiography.
2. Insert a pulmonary artery catheter for maximum safety and diagnostic information (see Chapter 3).
3. Explain the procedure to the patient and obtain consent.
4. Place the patient in the supine or 45° upright position. A 45° upright position might displace the pericardial cavity anteriorly, thereby reducing the distance from the anterior chest wall.
5. Wash your hands and put on sterile gown and gloves.
6. Prepare the patient by cleaning the lower, anterior chest wall and upper abdominal wall with povidone-iodine. Drape with sterile towels.
7. Infiltrate entry site with 2 to 10 mL of 1% lidocaine. The left subxiphoid approach is preferred, where the needle is inserted just to the left of the xiphoid process (Fig 6–1). An apical approach may also be used (fourth left intercostal space, parasternally).
8. Make a 2- to 3-mm skin incision.
9. Advance a long, large-bore needle (18 gauge) under the left subxiphoid region and direct it toward the

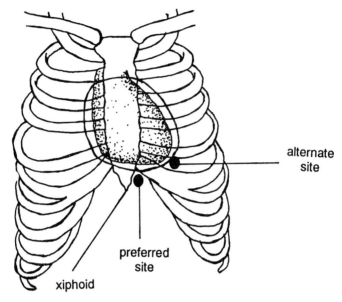

FIG 6–1.
The left subxiphoid approach for pericardiocentesis is preferred to avoid the major epicardial vessels and pleura. The apical location is an alternative site.

patient's left shoulder, at approximately 45°, while continuously aspirating. Alternatively, the needle may be directed toward the patient's head or right scapula. The needle may be flushed with the lidocaine contained in the syringe while advancing, providing additional anesthesia (Fig 6–2).

10. Attach an alligator clip to the distal portion of the needle and connect to the V lead of an EKG machine (Fig 6–3). Advance the needle as you monitor the intrapericardial EKG data. Direct contact with the right atrium or right ventricle is noted by PR or ST segment elevation, respectively. If epicardial contact is made, withdraw or reposition the needle. A promising new technique involves the use of a pacemaker attached to the pericardiocentesis needle. Epicardial contact is identified by the capture of the ventricle with the pacing stimulus. Appropriate grounding of these de-

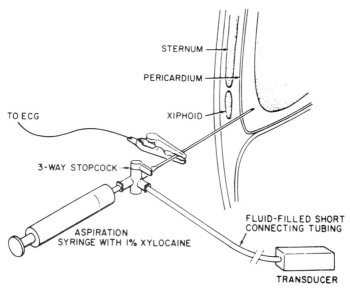

FIG 6-2.
The needle is attached to a syringe for continuous aspiration. The alligator clip is connected to the V lead of the EKG for the electrocardiographic assessment of needle location. Once fluid is obtained, the stopcock may be adjusted to record the pericardial pressure and its waveform via the fluid-filled connecting tube and a pressure transducer. (Modified from Lorell BH, Grossman W: Profiles in constrictive pericarditis, restrictive cardiomyopathy and cardiac tamponade. In Grossman W, Baim D, editors: *Cardiac catheterization, angiography and intervention,* ed 4, Philadelphia, 1986, Lea & Febiger, p 436. Used by permission.)

vices is essential, as ventricular fibrillation may be induced.

11. As the pericardial space is entered, you will notice a "popping" sensation followed by free aspiration of fluid. Place a clamp on the needle at the level of the skin to prevent inadvertent advancement. The pericardial pressure may be recorded at this step or at step 15.

12. With the Seldinger wire technique (Fig 6-4,A-D), insert the J-wire through the needle after removal of the syringe. Remove the needle. If fluoroscopy is available, position the wire into the posterior pericardial space.

13. Pass the dilator over the wire to dilate the track

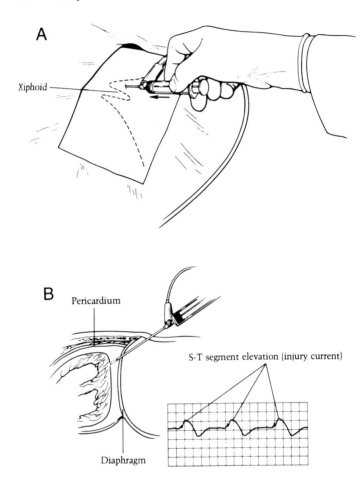

FIG 6–3.
The needle is inserted to the left of the xiphoid process **(A)** and advanced
while aspirating. The EKG is monitored closely while the needle is advanced. A current of injury (ST segment elevation) indicates epicardial
contact with the needle tip **(B)**. (From Ockene IS: Pericardiocentesis. In
Vander Salem TJ, Cutler BS, Wheeler HB (eds): *Atlas of bedside procedures,* ed 2, Boston, 1988, Little Brown, p 169. Used by permission.)

and then insert the pigtail catheter. A curved catheter
may also be used.

14. Connect the catheter to a stopcock and fluid-
filled pressure monitoring tubing.

15. Record pericardial pressures, preferably simulta-

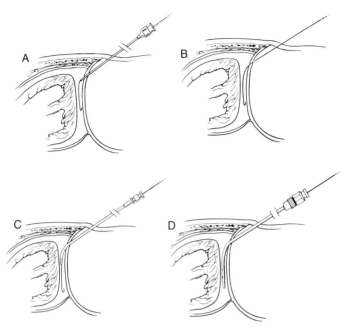

FIG 6–4.
Once the needle enters the pericardial space and fluid is withdrawn freely, a flexible J-tipped guidewire is advanced **(A)**. The needle is then removed, leaving the wire in place **(B)**. A dilator is slid over the guidewire and re-moved **(C)**. Finally, a short "pigtail" or curved catheter is advanced over the guidewire and positioned posteriorly **(D)**. The wire is then removed and the catheter is aspirated. Following the desired amount of fluid aspira-tion, the catheter may be sutured in placed, dressed, and remain in place for up to 48 hours for additional fluid withdrawal. (From Ockene IS: Peri-cardiocentesis. In Vander Salem TJ, Cutler BS, Wheeler HB (eds): *Atlas of bedside procedures,* ed 2, Boston, 1988, Little Brown, pp 172-173. Used by permission.)

neously with pressures from the right side of the heart.

16. Aspirate fluid with a 50-mL syringe or drainage bag. The multi-holed catheter prevents clogging.

17. Either suture the catheter in place or remove it after the drainage procedure.

18. Dress the insertion site.

19. Send specimens of pericardial fluid for analysis, including protein, glucose, amylase, white and red blood cell counts, hematocrit, Gram stain, and cultures (bacterial, fungal, acid-fast bacilli), cytology.

Additional Technical Recommendations

1. **Confirmation of needle/catheter position.** A small quantity of contrast material may be used to establish the position of the catheter. Swirling of the contrast material around the heart is a confirmatory sign of a pericardial location. Two-dimensional echocardiography also facilitates insertion of the needle into the appropriate location through identification of the closest region of fluid to the body wall and selection of the entry tract; this modality provides a success rate of 95% and no complications. The location of the needle/catheter may also be confirmed with contrast echocardiography.

2. *Pressure recording.* In elective circumstances, left and right heart catheterization are recommended in conjunction with pericardiocentesis for simultaneous pressure recordings of right ventricle/left ventricle, pericardium/right atrium, and pericardium/pulmonary artery occlusion pressure. Record pericardial pressure, systemic pressure, and pressure of the right side of the heart on entry into the pericardial space, after removal of 50 mL and 100 mL of fluid, and at the conclusion of procedure.

3. *Fluid removal.* Although confirmation of the pericardial source of sanguineous fluid is not always immediately possible, several clues often exist. The contracting heart causes defibrination of the blood; therefore, pericardial fluid should not clot. Clotted blood indicates inadvertent chamber puncture. Additionally, the hematocrit of the pericardial fluid should differ from that of peripheral blood. Clotting blood or a high hematocrit suggests cardiac chamber puncture.

Guidelines as to how much fluid to drain and how rapidly the effusion can be drained are unclear. Too rapid pericardial drainage can cause pulmonary edema, presumably because of a marked increase in ventricular filling while the systemic resistance remains elevated. It is recommended that enough pericardial fluid be removed to relieve tamponade and that, thereafter, the remaining pericardial effusion be drained gradually through the indwelling sidehole catheter. Removal of as little as 25 to 50 mL of fluid may result in dramatic hemodynamic improvement.

FOLLOW-UP

1. Following the procedure, obtain a chest roentgenogram to evaluate for a possible pneumothorax.

2. Observe the patient closely, with vital signs being checked every 15 minutes for the first several hours. The majority of patients should be monitored in an intensive care unit setting for a minimum of 24 hours.

3. A second echocardiogram is useful to document the effects of the pericardiocentesis and, if performed serially, to ensure there is no significant recurrence of the effusion.

4. Remove an indwelling pericardial catheter within 48 hours.

5. While pericardiocentesis may offer substantial diagnostic or therapeutic benefits, surgical intervention may still be required for definitive drainage, pericardial biopsy, or tumor resection.

COMPLICATIONS

1. Sometimes there is failure to obtain pericardial fluid. While not considered a true complication, a "dry" or nondiagnostic pericardiocentesis subjects the patient to substantial risk without significant benefit. Overall, the success rate of pericardiocentesis is greater than 80%, but may be much lower when posterior or small to moderate effusions are present or when hemopericardium is present with loculation. The more fluid, the less chance of a nonproductive tap or a complication. Therefore, despite the potential complications discussed later, pericardiocentesis can be performed with low risk in the majority of appropriately

selected patients, when the location and amount of pericardial fluid is accurately determined.

2. Mortality occurs in less than 5% of all pericardiocentesis procedures.
3. Cardiac chamber puncture, the most common complication (10%), is almost always without adverse sequelae. The right ventricle, right atria, and other cardiac chambers may be punctured inadvertently. Hemopericardium may occur but is not always associated with pericardial tamponade.
4. Arrhythmias may be caused by the irritation of ventricle or atrium by the needle or catheter.
5. Pulmonary edema, acute ventricular dilation, and volume overload might occur, probably secondary to a sudden increase in venous return on release of the tamponade.
6. Other described complications include the following.
   a. Laceration of coronary arteries.
   b. Pneumothorax.
   c. Perforation of abdominal viscus.
   d. Cardiac arrest.
   e. Vasovagal reactions.
   f. Infection.

DOCUMENTATION

Following completion of pericardiocentesis, a progress note entitled "Procedure Note—Pericardiocentesis" must be placed in the chart and signed by the operators. The following items should be included:

1. Indication for pericardiocentesis and elective or emergency designation.
2. Description of patient preparation and local anesthesia administered.
3. Choice of entry site and approach.
4. Use of EKG, fluoroscopic, or echocardiographic guidance.

5. Size and type of needle, dilator, and catheter.
6. Intracardiac and intrapericardial pressures.
7. Description and quantification of fluid removed.
8. Diagnostic studies ordered.
9. Complications encountered.

SUGGESTED READING

Bishop LH et al: The electrocardiogram as safeguard in pericardiocentesis, *JAMA* 62:254, 1956.

Callahan JA et al: Two-dimensional echocardiographically guided pericardiocentesis: experience in 117 consecutive patients, *Am J Cardiol* 55:476, 1985.

Kilpatrick ZM, Chapman CB: On pericardiocentesis, *Am J Cardiol* 16:722, 1965.

Krikorian JG, Hancock EW: Pericardiocentesis, *Am J Med* 65:808, 1978.

Lorell BH, Braunwald E: Pericardial disease. In Braunwald E editor: *Heart disease: a textbook of cardiovascular medicine*, ed 2, Philadelphia, 1988, WB Saunders.

Stewart JF, Gott VL: The use of a Seldinger wire technique for pericardiocentesis following cardiac surgery, *Ann Thorac Surg* 35:467, 1983.

Wong B et al: The risk of pericardiocentesis, *Am J Cardiol* 44:1110, 1979.

7

Apnea Testing for Determination of Brain Death

Roy D. Cane, M.B.B.Ch., F.F.A.,(S.A.)

INTRODUCTION

Determination of brain death depends on demonstration of irreversible cessation of all brain functions, including those mediated by the brain stem. Absence of the following reflexes is indicative of lack of brain stem function:

1. Pupillary reflex.
2. Oculocephalic reflex.
3. Oculovestibular reflex.
4. Corneal reflex.
5. Gag reflex.
6. Cough reflex.
7. Apnea.

OBJECTIVE

To determine whether the patient has a functioning intrinsic respiratory drive.

Indications

The patient manifests signs of brain death: is unresponsive to any stimulation, and is arreflexic and flaccid in the absence of central nervous system depressant and neuromuscular blocking drugs.

Contraindications

1. Presence of positive reflex activity for papillary, oculocephalic, oculovestibular, corneal, gag or cough reflexes.
2. Patient is receiving neuromuscular blocking drugs.
3. Patient is receiving central nervous system depressant drugs, especially those with a well-defined action on the respiratory center.

PREPARATION

Prior to performing apnea testing, consideration of the plan of action that will follow apnea testing is desirable. Questions that should be addressed include the following.

1. Is the patient a suitable candidate for organ donation?
2. Has organ donation been discussed with the patient's family or responsible agent?
3. Have decisions and appropriate orders been written regarding withdrawal of ventilatory support or re-institution of ventilatory support in the event that the patient is found to be apneic?

Equipment

A manual ventilator with oxygen source to deliver highest possible oxygen concentration is required.

Required Monitoring

1. Electrocardiogram.
2. Pulse oximeter.
3. Arterial blood gases.
4. Transcutaneous measurement of $PtcCO_2$ is an acceptable alternative to $Paco_2$ measurement.

Required Laboratory Data

Arterial blood gases.

PROCEDURE

The goal of apnea testing is to provide a maximal stimulus to the respiratory center and to evaluate whether a peripheral response to that stimulus results. Assuming that the patient's metabolic acid/base balance has been stable for at least 12 hours, blood and cerebrospinal fluid bicarbonate concentrations will be similar. As cerebrospinal fluid has only bicarbonate buffers, whereas blood has other buffers, the change in cerebrospinal fluid pH secondary to an acute increase in $Paco_2$ will be greater than that seen in the pH of the blood. An acute increase in $Paco_2$ of greater than 20 mm Hg can be expected to decrease the cerebrospinal fluid pH by approximately 0.2 unit. Available data suggest that an acute change in the pH of cerebral spinal fluid from a normal of approximately 7.35 to less than 7.20 will provide an adequate stimulus to the central respiratory chemoreceptor.

1. Place the patient on 100% oxygen for 5 minutes.
2. Establish continuous pulse oximetry and electrocardiogram monitoring.
3. Establish baseline blood pressure and heart rate.
4. Obtain baseline arterial blood gases.
5. Disconnect the patient from the ventilator and attach a manual ventilator with 100% oxygen source to the patient's airway.

6. Observe the patient very closely for any clinical evidence of spontaneous ventilatory efforts.

7. While closely monitoring pulse oximetric oxygen saturation (Spo_2), continue the apnea for 5 minutes to 6 minutes. The relationship between apnea time and measured $Paco_2$ in anesthetized patients is shown in Table 7–1. The rate of rise of $Paco_2$ will be determined by the patient's metabolic rate. Therefore, although the relationship between apnea time and $Paco_2$ is well documented, confirm in each patient that an appropriate stimulus has been achieved, as evidenced by an increase in $Paco_2$ of at least 20 mm Hg from baseline.

8. Repeat arterial blood gas analysis after 6 minutes of apnea. If the $Paco_2$ is more than 20 mm Hg higher than the baseline $Paco_2$, a reasonable apnea challenge has been performed. If the patient is still clinically apneic despite this increase in $Paco_2$, lack of brain stem function can be assumed.

9. Keep patients adequately oxygenated during an apnea challenge so that no iatrogenic damage to the patient is sustained, both for long-term purposes if the patient is found not to have brain death and for preservation of major organ function for potential organ donation. With preoxygenation on 100% oxygen, most patients will maintain an adequate Pao_2 during the

TABLE 7–1.

Predicted $Paco_2$-pH Relationships with Apneic Challenge*

Apnea Time (min)	$Paco_2$† (mm Hg)	pH (Units
0	40	7.400
1	52	7.340
2	55.5	7.323
3	59	7.305
4	62.5	7.288
5	66	7.260
10	83.5	7.183
15	101	7.095

*From Shapiro BA: The apnea–$Paco_2$ relationship: some clinical and medico-legal considerations, *J Clin Anesthesiol* 1:323–327, 1989. Used by permission.
†Arterial carbon dioxide pressure (tension).

TABLE 7–2.

Predicted Pa_{CO_2} Rate of Rise and pH Change in Apnea With One Positive Pressure Breath Every 30 Seconds*

Apnea Time (min)	Pa_{CO_2}† (mm Hg)	pH (Units
0	40	7.400
1	47	7.365
2	49.5	7.353
3	52	7.340
4	54.5	7.328
5	57	7.315
10	69.5	7.253
15	82	7.190

*From Shapiro BA: The apnea–Pa_{CO_2} relationship: some clinical and medico-legal considerations, *J Clin Anesthesiol* 1:323–327, 1989. Used by permission.
†Arterial carbon dioxide tension.

period of apnea. However, during the apneic challenge, if the arterial saturation falls below 90%, ventilate the patient and restore the alveolar Po_2 and hence arterial oxygenation. Ventilation will reduce the rate of rise of Pa_{CO_2} and mandate a longer apnea challenge. The relationship between apnea time and Pa_{CO_2} when the patient is given a single positive pressure breath every 30 seconds is shown in Table 7–2.

If the Sa_{O_2} falls below 90%, ventilate the patient manually with four or five large inflations until the Sa_{O_2} increases to greater than 90%. Thereafter, give a single manual breath every 30 seconds. Achievement of an appropriate apneic challenge under these circumstances usually requires a period of apneic challenge of approximately 10 minutes. After 10 minutes, check arterial blood gases to ensure that the Pa_{CO_2} has risen by at least 20 mm Hg.

FOLLOW-UP

The decisions regarding withdrawal or continuance of cardiopulmonary support and organ donation will determine the follow-up steps to be taken.

COMPLICATIONS

Development of significant arterial desaturation ($Spo_2 < 90\%$) during apnea is the only complication. If the patient does not maintain adequate arterial oxygenation during apnea, it is necessary to provide an occasional positive pressure breath with pure oxygen to support arterial oxygenation. As discussed, this will mandate a longer apneic challenge to achieve an appropriate result.

DOCUMENTATION

The procedure note should include:

1. Findings of the clinical examination and discussions that lead to performance of an apneic challenge.
2. The preapneic and postapneic challenge arterial blood gases.
3. The patient's arterial oxygen saturation and blood pressure values during the apneic challenge.

SUGGESTED READING

Shapiro BA: The apnea-$Paco_2$ relationship: some clinical and medico-legal considerations, *J Clin Anesthesiol* 1:323–327, 1989.

Stock MC et al: The $Paco_2$ rate of rise in anesthetized patients with airway obstruction, *J Clin Anesthesiol* 1:328–32, 1989.

8

Volume Loading

Richard Davison, M.D.

INTRODUCTION

Maintenance of an adequate intravascular volume is essential for optimal function of the cardiovascular system. With critical illness, many factors conspire to alter cardiovascular homeostasis. Measurements of blood volume can be performed with reasonable accuracy at the bedside, but the technique is burdensome and does not lend itself to the serial measurements required by a rapidly changing situation. Alternatively, ventricular volumes can be quantitated and used as a reflection of the degree of diastolic filling which, in turn, depends on the adequacy of the blood volume. Unfortunately, this technique is also plagued with difficulties. The current method of volume loading usually used for the evaluation and "on-line" monitoring of intravascular volume includes all of the following components:

1. Accurate measurement of the filling pressures of the heart.
2. Assessment of the response of the filling pressures to a sudden, transient increase in venous return.

3. Evaluation of the changes produced by this maneuver on other physiological and/or clinical parameters.

OBJECTIVE

The primary therapeutic purpose of volume loading is to restore the intravascular volume to a level consistent with optimal cardiovascular function.

Within limits, volume loading also can provide important diagnostic information, both on the state of intravascular volume and on the degree of compliance of the ventricles.

Indications

1. If the adequacy of the intravascular volume is in doubt.
2. When low venous pressure is believed to have resulted in inadequate diastolic filling. Restoration of diastolic filling may improve stroke volume.

Contraindications

Volume loading should not be attempted if

1. Clinical or hemodynamic parameters suggest intravascular plethora.
2. The attendant increase in filling pressures could pose a risk to the patient, such as impending pulmonary edema.

PREPARATION

Venous access is necessary for the administration of intravenous fluids. A large-bore central venous line is preferred, though any venous catheter can be used. See

Chapter 2 for information regarding placement of a central venous catheter.

Equipment

Intravenous fluid for volume expansion is required, either

1. Crystalloid fluid, such as normal saline, or Ringer's lactate.
2. Colloid solution, such as hetastarch or albumin.

The technique to be followed for safe volume loading is not significantly influenced by the characteristics of the expanding agent chosen; therefore, volume expansion fluids will not be discussed here.

Required Monitoring

The extent of monitoring required will depend on

1. The degree of accuracy with which the baseline filling pressures need to be ascertained.
2. The parameter or parameters chosen to evaluate the results of volume loading.

Useful monitors include the following.

1. Clinical parameters of cardiac function.
   a. Heart rate.
   b. Arterial blood pressure. In instances where a hypovolemic state is clinically obvious and there is no indication of pre-existing cardiac or pulmonary disease, assessment of the response of the heart rate and arterial blood pressure (and their postural changes) to volume replacement will suffice.
2. Hemodynamic pressure monitors.
   a. Pulmonary artery catheter. When the initial volume status is uncertain, especially if the

situation is obscured by a concurrent disease process, intravascular monitoring with a flow-directed pulmonary artery catheter becomes mandatory. The pulmonary artery occluded pressure (PAOP) will most often be the parameter used to estimate the baseline status of the intravascular volume.

b. Central venous pressure (CVP). Right atrial pressures become equally important in specific instances, which include the following.

   (1) Acute cor pulmonale, such as pulmonary embolism.

   (2) Right ventricular myocardial infarction.

   (3) Cardiac tamponade.

3. Parameters of tissue perfusion. Besides the response of the PAOP/CVP to volume loading, a variety of additional endpoints can be used to assess the results of this intervention.

   a. Clinical parameters.

      (1) Urine output.

      (2) Skin temperature.

      (3) Mental status.

   b. Hemodynamic parameters.

      (1) Cardiac output/index.

      (2) Blood pressure.

      (3) Heart rate.

   c. Metabolic parameters.

      (1) Arteriovenous oxygen content difference.

      (2) Mixed venous blood oxygen saturation.

      (3) Arterial pH.

      (4) Serum lactate concentration.

Required Laboratory Data

None.

PROCEDURE

Measurement of PAOP with a pulmonary artery catheter is probably the most common monitor employed for volume loading; thus, this discussion will focus on volume loading with PAOP monitoring. The same procedure can be followed using any of the other indices of cardiovascular performance listed earlier instead of the PAOP.

1. Establish the baseline PAOP. Interpretation of the initial PAOP is fairly straightforward **only if the PAOP is low.** In all other circumstances, the following variables must be considered.
   a. If the patient is receiving positive-end-expiratory pressure (PEEP) of more than 5 cm of water, the PAOP may be factitiously elevated by transmitted positive intrathoracic pressure. No accurate way exists to assess in any individual patient the degree to which a particular level of PEEP contributes to the PAOP.
   b. Under normal circumstances, the spontaneous filling pressure of the left ventricle is regulated very close to the level where it provides optimal end-diastolic volumes. Attempts at "overfilling" a normal left ventricle may result in a relatively small gain in stroke volume associated with a significant rise in PAOP (Fig 8–1, curve A).
   c. An elevated initial PAOP is not a contraindication to an attempt at volume loading in the presence of an abnormal left ventricle. For example, in the setting of acute myocardial infarction, a PAOP below 18 mm Hg usually results in suboptimal filling of the left ventricle. Similarly, the enlarged ventricle found in congestive heart failure functions best at considerably elevated PAOP.
2. Administer 100 to 200 mL of fluid intravenously over 10 to 15 minutes.
3. Repeat measurement of PAOP. Possible outcomes and recommended actions are summarized in Table 8–1.

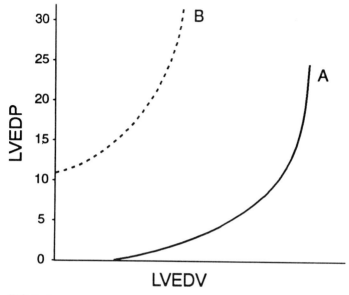

FIG 8–1.
Schematic diagram of left ventricular pressure/volume curves: *A* = normal ventricle. *B* = ventricle with reduced compliance.

A prompt and significant increase in PAOP (5 mm Hg or greater) suggests that intravascular volume and venous return are adequate and/or that left ventricular compliance is limited. Regardless of the underlying mechanism, further loading will only result in a mod-

TABLE 8–1.
Possible Outcomes From Volume Loading

Pulmonary Artery Occluded Pressure	Endpoint	Action
Unchanged	Unchanged	Continue VE*
Unchanged	Improved	Continue VE
Decreased	Improved	Continue VE
Increased (≤5 mm Hg)	Improved	Continue cautious VE
Increased (≤5 mm Hg)	Unchanged	Continue cautious VE
Markedly increased (>5 mm Hg)	Unchanged	Discontinue VE

*VE = volume expansion.

est increase in end diastolic volume at best (see Fig 8–1).

Occasionally, volume loading paradoxically decreases PAOP. The hemodynamic sequence behind this phenomenon is as follows. An increase in venous return improves left ventricular end diastolic volume, which in turn results in a greater stroke volume. As flow improves, systemic vascular resistance decreases, leading to a reduction in left ventricular afterload. This will improve systolic emptying and reduce end diastolic volume, which will be reflected in a decrease in PAOP.

Volume Loading Without Hemodynamic Pressure Monitoring

Follow essentially the same procedure as when a pulmonary catheter is in place.

1. Establish baseline values of the clinical signs that reflect cardiovascular performance.
2. Administer fluid load.
3. Reassess clinical signs of cardiovascular performance.
4. If no improvement is noted in cardiovascular performance after administration of several fluid challenges or if patient develops clinical signs suggestive of pulmonary edema, it is wise to consider placement of a pulmonary artery catheter to enable more accurate assessment of cardiovascular performance.

FOLLOW-UP

Table 8–2 is a list of the recommended actions following initial volume expansion. It is not unusual for the PAOP to slowly decrease after the initial rise. This decrease is due either to subsequent vasodilatation or to diffusion of fluid out of the intravascular space. If the hemodynamic improvement that had been achieved is noted to regress, further volume loading will be re-

TABLE 8–2.

Follow-up After Initial Volume Loading

Pulmonary Artery Occluded Pressure	Endpoint	Action
Drifts down	Worsens	Increased volume administration
Drifts down	Remains good	Fluid administration at maintenance level
Drifts up	Remains good	Decreased volume administration
Drifts up	Worsens	Add another therapy

quired to restore PAOP. Conversely, if despite the decrease in PAOP the hemodynamic advantage persists, continued observation is advised before the fluid challenge is repeated.

When the PAOP continues to rise after the initial fluid challenge, several possibilities need to be considered.

1. Excessive fluid may have been administered.
2. Ventricular function may be deteriorating.
3. A pericardial tamponade may be present.
4. Venous return may have increased secondary to the following.
   a. Withdrawal of positive pressure ventilation.
   b. Reabsorption of "third space" fluid.
   c. Discontinuation of vasodilator medication.

COMPLICATIONS

1. Intravascular volume overload.
2. Pulmonary edema.

DOCUMENTATION

Use of a flowsheet listing the PAOP, endpoint parameters, and volume administration is essential to proper interpretation of the initial and subsequent responses to volume loading. On completion of adequate fluid loading, write a procedure note that includes the following:

1. Indication for fluid loading.
2. Baseline parameters of cardiovascular performance.
3. Nature and volume of fluid administered.
4. Cardiovascular response to fluid loading.
5. Any complications that may have occurred.

SUGGESTED READING

Calvin JE et al: Does the pulmonary capillary wedge pressure predict left ventricular pre-load in critically ill patients?, *Crit Care Med* 9:437, 1981.

Crexels C et al: Optimal level of ventricular filling pressure in the left side of the heart in acute myocardial infraction, *N Engl J Med* 289:1263, 1973.

Jardin F et al: Influence of positive and end-expiratory pressure on left ventricular performance, *N Engl J Med* 304:387, 1981.

Parker JO, Case RB: Normal left ventricular function, *Circulation* 60:4, 1979.

9

Oxygen Challenge

Roy D. Cane, M.B.B.Ch., F.F.A.(S.A.)

INTRODUCTION

Hypoxemia, defined as an arterial oxygen tension (Pa_{O_2}) of less than 80 mm Hg when room air is being breathed, develops as a result of changes in pulmonary parenchymal function, cardiac function, and tissue oxygen utilization. In simplistic terms, hypoxemia secondary to pulmonary disease can be conceptualized as a consequence of alterations in ventilation-perfusion ratio relationships ($\dot{V}/\dot{Q}$). In an alveolar-capillary unit with a $\dot{V}/\dot{Q}$ ratio of 1, complete saturation of the hemoglobin will be achieved (Fig 9–1,A). In an alveolar-capillary unit with a $\dot{V}/\dot{Q}$ of 0 (shunt unit), no change will occur in the oxyhemoglobin saturation of the blood (Fig 9–1,B). Blood passing through alveolar-capillary units with $\dot{V}/\dot{Q}$ of greater than 0, but less than 1 (venous admixture unit), will be partially saturated (Fig 9–1,C). The oxyhemoglobin saturation of blood in the left atrium is determined by the mix of blood from all three forms of $\dot{V}/\dot{Q}$ units. When lung disease results in an increase in the relative amount of lung with $\dot{V}/\dot{Q}$ relationships less than 1, the net effect is arterial hypoxemia.

Figure 9–2 illustrates the effect of breathing 100% oxygen on the hypoxemia associated with venous ad-

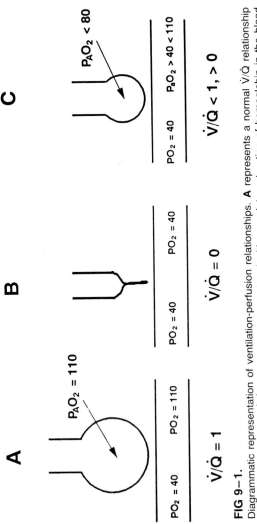

FIG 9–1.
Diagrammatic representation of ventilation-perfusion relationships. **A** represents a normal $\dot{V}/\dot{Q}$ relationship with a ratio of 1. This $\dot{V}/\dot{Q}$ relationship is associated with complete saturation of hemoglobin in the blood passing through this alveolar-capillary unit. **B** represents a shunt unit ($\dot{V}/\dot{Q} = 0$). The oxyhemoglobin saturation of blood passing through this unit is unchanged. **C** represents an alveolar-capillary unit with a $\dot{V}/\dot{Q}$ of < 1, but > 0. Hemoglobin in the blood passing through this unit is only partially saturated.

mixture. Alveolus A represents a venous admixture unit ($\dot{V}/\dot{Q} < 1$ but > 0), whereas alveolus B is normal ($\dot{V}/\dot{Q} = 1$). Denitrogenation associated with breathing 100% oxygen increases the partial pressure of oxygen in the alveoli (Pao$_2$) in the underventilated alveolus to a level sufficient to ensure complete oxyhemoglobin saturation of the blood, thereby hypoxemia is corrected. To

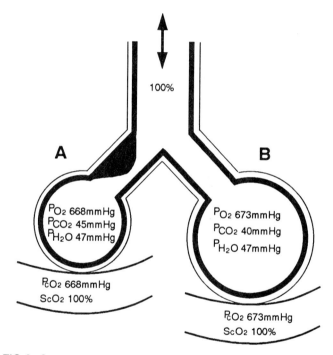

FIG 9–2.
Diagrammatic representation of the effect of breathing 100% oxygen on hypoxemia caused by venous admixture. Alveolus *A* represents a unit with normal perfusion but diminished ventilation ($\dot{V}/\dot{Q}$ of < 1, > 0); alveolus *B* represents a unit with normal perfusion and ventilation ($\dot{V}/\dot{Q} = 1$). The alveolar and pulmonary capillary gas tensions and oxyhemoglobin saturations reflect ideal values when an individual is breathing 100% oxygen. Denitrogenation secondary to breathing 100% oxygen results in no significant differences in the P$_{AO_2}$ and P$_{CO_2}$ between alveolar-capillary units. (From Limitations of oxygen therapy. In Shapiro BA et al: *Clinical application of respiratory care,* ed 4, St Louis, 1989, Mosby–Year Book, p 137. Used by permission.)

achieve complete oxyhemoglobin saturation of blood passing an alveolus requires a P_{AO_2} greater than 80 mm Hg. The fraction of inspired oxygen (FI_{O_2}) needed to elevate P_{AO_2} above 80 mm Hg depends on the magnitude of $\dot{V}/\dot{Q}$ discrepancy; the lower the $\dot{V}/\dot{Q}$, the higher the required FI_{O_2}. For practical purposes, hypoxemia secondary to venous admixture is responsive to oxygen therapy and is usually corrected with FI_{O_2} up to 0.5.

Hypoxemia caused by shunt mechanisms is barely responsive to increased inspired oxygen concentrations. The blood passing through shunt units is not exposed to alveolar air; therefore, it is unaffected by an increase in alveolar oxygen tensions. Alveolar oxygen tensions in the undiseased lung are usually greater than 80 mm Hg in room air conditions; therefore, little additional oxygen can be added to the exposed blood by an increase in these alveolar oxygen tensions. Thus the hypoxemia associated with shunt mechanisms can be characterized as being refractory to oxygen therapy. The possibility that a refractory hypoxemia is present should be considered when the Pa_{O_2} is less than 55 mm Hg on a FI_{O_2} greater than 0.35.

Most hypoxemias result from combinations of shunt and venous admixture mechanisms. Because concentrations of inspired oxygen above 50% are potentially harmful, identifying hypoxemic states that are relatively refractory to oxygen therapy is important. The oxygen challenge is a useful clinical technique that helps to differentiate between those patients with refractory hypoxemia (predominantly caused by shunt) from those that are adequately responsive to oxygen therapy (predominantly caused by venous admixture).

OBJECTIVE

Identify those patients with hypoxemia predominantly caused by shunt mechanisms in whom support of arterial oxygenation requires more than oxygen therapy.

Indications

Severe hypoxemia, as evidenced by a Pa_{O_2} of less than 55 mm Hg on a F_{IO_2} between 0.21 and 0.35.

Contraindications

Hypoxemia in patients with chronic obstructive pulmonary disease associated with chronic alveolar hypoventilation; these patients may hypoventilate further in response to hyperoxia.

PREPARATION

Equipment

High-flow oxygen-delivery system capable of delivering a reliable F_{IO_2} between 0.21 and 0.5.

Required Monitoring

None.

Required Laboratory Data

Arterial blood gas (ABG) analysis.

PROCEDURE

1. Explain to the patient that you are going to test the response of his/her Pa_{O_2} to increases in inspired oxygen concentration.
2. Obtain ABG analysis after the patient has been undisturbed on baseline F_{IO_2} (ideally between 0.21 to 0.35) for at least 30 minutes.
3. Increase F_{IO_2} by 0.2, which, in theory, will result in an increase in Pa_{O_2} of approximately 90 mm Hg at sea level.
4. Wait 15 to 30 minutes for the alveolar oxygen ten-

sions to stabilize on the higher F_{IO_2} and repeat the ABG analysis.

5. If the Pa_{O_2} increases less than 10 mm Hg, the primary pathophysiology responsible for the hypoxemia is most likely a shunt mechanism. Figure 9–3 illustrates the oxygen challenge for two patients with a baseline Pa_{O_2} of 40 mm Hg on a F_{IO_2} of 0.21. "Patient A" has a hypoxemia caused by a large shunt (30%) with a small component of venous admixture. "Patient B" has a hypoxemia caused by a small shunt (15%) with a large component of venous admixture.

6. Seek the possible cause of refractory hypoxemia. The most common conditions that produce refractory hypoxemia are listed in Table 9–1. These disease pro-

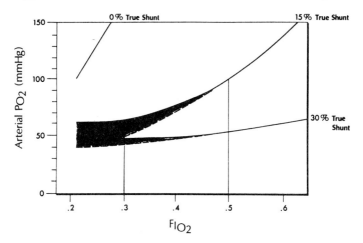

FIG 9–3.
Representation of two patients with a Pa_{O_2} of 40 mm Hg breathing room air. Patient A's hypoxemia is due to a 30% shunt with a small additional component of venous admixture. Patient B's hypoxemia is due to a shunt of 15% with a large additional component of venous admixture. The *broken lines* represent the Pa_{O_2}-F_{IO_2} relationships from both the shunt and venous admixture, whereas, the *solid lines* represent the Pa_{O_2}-F_{IO_2} relationships from the shunt alone. The oxygen challenge, increasing F_{IO_2} from 0.3 to 0.5, results in an increase in Pa_{O_2} of < 10 mm Hg for patient A (refractory hypoxemia) and of > 10 mm Hg for patient B (responsive hypoxemia). (From Limitations of oxygen therapy. In Shapiro BA et al: *Clinical application of respiratory care*, ed 4, St Louis, 1991, Mosby–Year Book, p 141. Used by permission.)

TABLE 9–1.

Common Disease Conditions
Producing Refractory Hypoxemia*

Cardiovascular
  Right-to-left intracardiac shunt
  Pulmonary arteriovenous fistula
Pulmonary
  Consolidated pneumonitis
  Lobar atelectasis
  Large neoplasm
  Adult respiratory distress
    syndrome

*From Shapiro BA et al: Oxygen therapy.
In *Clinical application of respiratory care*,
ed 4, St Louis, 1991, Mosby–Year Book.
Used by permission.

cesses usually can be differentiated by careful clinical
history, physical examination, and chest roentgenogram after oxygen challenge indicates that a refractory
hypoxemia exists.

COMPLICATIONS

None.

DOCUMENTATION

Write a note in the chart that reflects the following:

1. Baseline Pa_{O_2} and F_{IO_2}.
2. Oxygen challenge F_{IO_2} and resultant increase in
Pa_{O_2}.
3. Interpretation of result of oxygen challenge: hypoxemia, refractory, or responsive.
4. Differential diagnosis of disease process responsible for the hypoxemia.
5. Plan for further diagnostic steps.
6. Therapeutic plan for support of the patient's arterial oxygenation.

SUGGESTED READING

Davidson FF et al: The components of the alveolar-arterial oxygen tension difference in normal subjects and in patients with pneumonia and obstructive lung disease, *Am J Med* 52:754, 1972.

Shapiro BA et al: Hypoxemia and oxygen therapy. In *Clinical application of blood gases*, ed 4, St Louis, 1989, Mosby–Year Book.

10

Bronchoscopy

Kenneth L. Holling, M.D.
Michael D. Hammond, M.D.

INTRODUCTION

The development of fiberoptic bronchoscopy for the diagnosis and treatment of pulmonary disease has significantly advanced the quality of care provided to critically ill patients. The fiberoptic bronchoscope, developed in the 1960s by Shigeto Ikeda, revolutionized the practice of pulmonary medicine. Fiberoptic bronchoscopy has not only evolved into the most important method of evaluating local and diffuse lung disease, but also become important therapeutically in the management of critically ill ventilated patients.

OBJECTIVES

1. To aid in the diagnosis of pulmonary disease in critically ill patients.
2. To facilitate bronchial hygiene therapy in critically ill patients with pulmonary disease.

Indications

The American Thoracic Society recognizes varied diagnostic and therapeutic indications for fiberoptic bronchoscopy (Table 10–1). Additional recommendations include the following.

1. Bronchoscopy should not be employed routinely as a substitute for conventional noninvasive techniques for mobilizing pulmonary secretions.
2. Bronchoscopy is not routinely necessary in obtaining sputum for diagnostic study in cases of pneumonia or acute bronchitis.

Contraindications

In a consenting patient, no absolute contraindications to fiberoptic bronchoscopy exist; however, several conditions increase the risk of complications. Proper patient selection and careful consideration of the risks and benefits are essential. A list of the relative contraindications to fiberoptic bronchoscopy, as outlined by the American Thoracic Society, is shown in Table 10–2.

TABLE 10–1.

Indications for Fiberoptic Bronchoscopy

Diagnostic
   Evaluation of diffuse or focal abnormalities seen on the chest
      roentgenogram
   Tissue collection for pathologic and microbiological evaluation
   Hemoptysis
   Assessment of endotracheal tube placement
   Assessment of the airways
      Patency
      Bronchial fracture after chest trauma
      Inhalation/burn injury
      Evaluation for aspiration of gastric contents
Therapeutic
   Removal of mucus plugs causing atelectasis
   Removal of foreign bodies
   Difficult intubation

TABLE 10–2.

Contraindications and Risks in Fiberoptic Bronchoscopy

Risk conditions
  Poor patient cooperation
  Recent myocardial infarction; unstable angina
  Partial tracheal obstruction
  Unstable asthma
  Hepatitis
  Uremia and pulmonary hypertension
  Lung abscess
  Immunosuppression
  Superior vena cava obstruction
  Respiratory insufficiency with refractory hypoxemia or acute
    hypercapnia, debility, advanced age, malnutrition
High-risk conditions
  Malignant arrhythmias
  Profound refractory hypoxemia
  Severe bleeding diathesis that cannot be corrected when biopsy
    procedure is anticipated

PREPARATION

Training

Proper training in patient preparation, bronchoscopic technique, and handling of specimens is essential to optimize patient safety and diagnostic yield. The physician appropriately trained in bronchoscopy will be able to fulfill the following.

1. Describe normal bronchial anatomy.
2. Identify indications and contraindications for bronchoscopy.
3. Determine when rigid or flexible instruments should be used.
4. Identify and state the purpose of each tool (for example, a specimen collector), its capabilities, and when each should be used.
5. Anticipate possible complications of flexible bronchoscopy and conditions associated with each complication.

6. Select the appropriate premedication and write orders before and after bronchoscopy.

7. Describe the bronchoscopy procedure in lay terms.

8. Intubate (endotracheal) using the flexible bronchoscope.

9. Maintain a patent, adequate airway at all times.

10. Introduce a flexible bronchoscope by the transnasal, transoral, and tracheostomy routes.

11. Complete an endoscopic inspection of the entire tracheobronchial tree and direct the tip of the bronchoscope into any given segment of the tracheobronchial tree.

12. Carry out the following diagnostic techniques: bronchial brushing, forceps biopsy including transbronchial lung biopsy, and segmental bronchoalveolar lavage.

13. Manage complications as they arise.

14. Properly clean and maintain bronchoscopic equipment.

Equipment

The most efficient way to keep needed equipment immediately available is to maintain a cart stocked with a wide variety of supplies. Table 10–3 lists an example of a well-stocked bronchoscopy cart.

Bronchoscopes are either rigid and flexible. Although the most commonly used are the flexible fiberoptic bronchoscopes, the two are interchangeable for many indications. However, in some circumstances a specific type of bronchoscope is recommended. The fiberoptic bronchoscope is the instrument of choice when bronchoscopy is needed for patients on mechanical ventilators or for those with disease or trauma involving the skull, jaws, or cervical spine; the rigid open-tube bronchoscope is the instrument of choice during massive hemoptysis.

Several brands and models of flexible fiberoptic bronchoscopes are available. These differ little in basic

TABLE 10−3.

Equipment for Bronchoscopy Cart

Bronchoscope and teaching head	Cetacaine spray
Light source	Glass slides
Video equipment (optional)	Formalin containers
Suction device	Cytology fixative spray and
Lidocaine, 1% and 2%	container
Viscous lidocaine	Sterile normal saline
Sponge; 4 × 4 gauze	Assortment of endotracheal tubes;
Assortment of needles and	oral intubator
syringes	Swivel tube adaptors
Atomizer	Ambu bag
Oxygen supplies	Suction tubing and tubing
Assortment of biopsy forceps	connectors
Aspiration needles	Gloves, masks, and gowns
Cytology brushes	Epinephrine
Protected brushes	Atropine, 1-mg vial
Pathology, cytology, and	Beta agonist, unit dose
microbiology request forms	Intravenous supplies
Bronchoscopy procedure reports	Oral intubator

design; however, the models differ considerably according to the specific function for which they were designed.

The basic bronchoscope consists of a control unit and a shaft. The control unit is made up of the viewport, optics, and a control lever that deflects the distal tip of the shaft. The control unit also contains the wall suction port and a port continuous with the working channel. In some models, occlusion of the working port effects suction at the distal tip. In newer models, the working port is offset from the suction actuator. The flexible shaft is marked at 5-cm intervals. The content of the shaft include guidewires for deflection of the tip, efferent and afferent glass fiber bundles, and the working channel.

Bronchoscopes are classified as pediatric, standard adult, therapeutic, photodocumentation, and video bronchoscopes. They vary in view angle, tip deflection, shaft diameter, working channel diameter, and shaft length. Therapeutic bronchoscopes have the largest working port diameter for easy removal of secretions, while the standard adult bronchoscope has a slim shaft for patient comfort. The shaft diameter is also important when the endotracheal tube route is used; however, photodocumentation bronchoscopes, which have a large shaft diameter, sacrifice working channel diameter for improved optics.

A comprehensive range of therapeutic accessories is available for the bronchoscope. Standard and ellipsoid biopsy forceps are fenestrated to reduce crush artifact. Fenestrated, ellipsoid forceps with a terminal spike are used to impale and stabilize the forceps on a "slippery" lesion. Forceps with alligator teeth are used in biopsy procedures on tough tissue. These forceps have stainless steel jaws and are autoclavable.

Brushes are used for cytologic and microbiologic collection purposes. The designs vary, but are of two basic types: (1) unsheathed, disposable cytology brushes, and (2) sheathed, reusable brushes designed to reduce contamination and specimen loss.

A variety of retrieval forceps are designed to grasp various foreign bodies. Rat-tooth forceps are suited for grasping coins and flat objects, while a three-pronged forceps is suited for grasping chunks of necrotic tissue. Rubber-tipped forceps are used to grasp sharp objects such as pins and needles, and a magnetic probe is used to remove ferrous objects. A retractable four-filament basket is suited for retrieving larger objects.

Retractable 21-gauge, 13-mm needles are used for transbronchial aspiration, and smaller injection needles are available. Other specialty items include bronchial catheters, balloon-tipped occlusion catheters, and curettes.

Required Monitoring

1. Pulse oximetry.
2. Continuous electrocardiographic monitoring.

Required Laboratory Data

1. Thorough review of the chest roentgenogram is essential to guide the bronchoscopist to the area in which to focus the procedure.

2. In critically ill patients, an arterial blood gas analysis is frequently needed to assess the degree of hypoxemia and hypercapnia.

3. A PT and PTT are necessary if a biopsy is anticipated and the possibility of a bleeding diathesis exists.

4. Additional data may be required depending on the clinical circumstances.

PROCEDURE

1. Thoroughly review the indications for the procedure, its risks, the chest roentgenogram, and the current endotracheal tube size (if the patient is intubated).

2. Approach the patient or family and explain the procedure.

3. Relieve anxiety.

4. Obtain informed consent.

5. Write orders, as appropriate. The patient should neither eat nor drink for 8 hours, if possible, prior to the procedure.

6. Thirty minutes prior to the procedure, premedicate the patient with atropine, 0.8 to 1.0 mg intramuscularly. Beneficial effects of atropine include reduction of secretions, blocking of the vasovagal reflex, and bronchodilation. Alert patients require sedation; meperidine, 50 to 150 mg, or morphine, 5 to 15 mg intramuscularly, is recommended because narcotics are reversible with naloxone. The dosages should be adjusted according to the patient's weight, age, and condition. Benzodiazipines, such as Valium (diazepam), 5 mg intravenously, are frequently used when additional sedation is needed. Caution should be used to avoid oversedation and hypoventilation.

7. Ensure that the indicated precautions to reduce the patient's risk are being taken, such as pulse oximetry, cardiac monitoring, use of preprocedure beta-agonist. (See Complications.)

8. In ventilated patients, preoxygenate with 100% oxygen. Because auto–positive end-expiratory pressure (PEEP) can develop when the effective cross-sectional area of the endotrachial tube is reduced by the bronchoscope, monitor the PEEP, keeping it below 20 cm of water. In nonventilated patients, administer supplemental oxygen by nasal cannula.

9. The bronchoscopist and assistant should wear gowns, gloves, masks, and eye protection.

10. The patient is asked to sit, or is positioned with the head of the bed elevated 30°.

11. Attach a swivel adapter, with cap in place, to the endotracheal tube or tracheostomy cannula and connect to the ventilator tubing. This adapter minimizes loss of tidal volume.

12. Ventilated patients who are alert, or who cough with routine suctioning, require topical anesthesia. Inject 3 to 5 mL of 1% or 2% lidocaine through the swivel adapter and into the tracheobronchial tree. Alternatively, administer lidocaine by an in-line aerosol. Further anesthesia can be administered through the working port of the bronchoscope during the procedure as needed. Anesthesia of the upper airway can be accomplished in nonventilated patients with 3 mL of 2% lidocaine sprayed into the nose and posterior oropharynx or with 2% lidocaine soaked on a cotton swab and inserted into the nose. Other techniques for anesthesia include 30 mL of lidocaine used as a gargle or application of lidocaine-soaked cotton balls to each pyriform sinus for 1 minute. The patient can be asked to sniff 3 mL of lidocaine jelly into the nasal passage for additional anesthesia and lubrication.

13. Choose the proper bronchoscope after considering patient comfort, endotrachal tube size, and purpose of the procedure (diagnostic or therapeutic). After appropriate connections to the suction and light source

are made, pass the lubricated bronchoscope into the tracheobronchial tree through a tracheostomy or endotracheal tube. When an endotracheal tube is used, its position in relation to the carina should be evaluated. In nonintubated patients, pass the lubricated bronchoscope into the hypopharynx by way of the transnasal or transoral route. Apply additional anesthesia to the vocal cords under direct vision through the working port of the bronchoscope. Carefully inspect the larynx and vocal cords. Evaluate vocal cord mobility by having the patient say "E."

14. In patients on ventilators, adjust the tidal volume to compensate for volume loss through the swivel adapter and from suctioning. Adjust airway pressure limits to compensate for increased airway resistance caused by decreased airway cross-sectional area.

15. A rapid, yet complete, survey of the airways is then undertaken. Start with the area that is not the focus of the procedure. Then turn your attention to the area in which the remainder of the procedure is to take place.

16. Retained secretions and mucus plugs can be mobilized with 5- to 30-mL boluses of sterile isotonic saline injected through the working port into the tracheobronchial tree under direct vision, then removed with suction. Use a therapeutic bronchoscope with a 2.8-mm working channel. The total irrigation fluid should not exceed 300 mL.

17. Endobronchial anatomy is shown in Figure 10–1. Findings associated with malignancy include a fixed or splayed main carina or subcarina, external airway compression or airway distortion, localized mucosal inflammation or cobblestone appearance, and an endobronchial mass or ulceration. Signs of acute bronchial inflammation include purulent secretions, longitudinal ridges, and mucosal erythema and edema. Signs of chronic inflammation include copious secretion, transverse muscular banding, and mucus gland ductal ectasia.

18. When abnormalities are visualized in the bron-

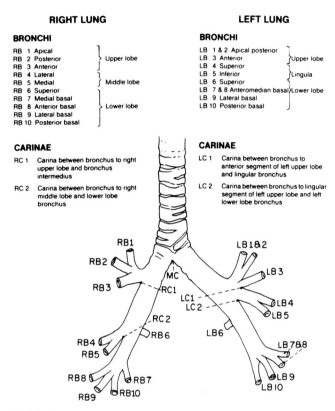

FIG 10–1.
Endobronchial anatomy. *MC* = main carina; *RB* = right bronchus; *LB* = left bronchus; *RC* = right carina; *LC* = left carina. (From Prakash UB, Fontana RS: Functional classification of bronchial carinae, *Chest* 86:770, 1984. Used by permission.)

chi, obtain endobronchial forceps biopsy and brushings. Pass the forceps through the working port and into the bronchi. Acquiring samples of lesions directly ahead of the bronchoscope for biopsy examination is not difficult, and larger, stiffer forceps can be used. When a lesion is in an upper lobe, requiring sharp angulation, a smaller flexible forceps shaft is desirable. When a lesion is on a lateral wall, use a spiked forceps to impale the lesion and stabilize the forceps prior to taking a biopsy sample. Two to three milliliters of a

1:10,000 solution of epinephrine can be applied as a bolus to a tumor to prevent excessive bleeding prior to biopsy.

A cytologic brush can be repeatedly passed over a lesion to collect cells and tissue fragments. Ideally, the brush should be sheathed while being passed in and out of the working channel of the bronchoscope, and exposed only in the bronchi. Doing so prevents loss of biopsy material. The diagnostic yield of brushings in central, visible, bronchogenic carcinomas is 94%; however, the diagnostic yield is poor in cases of alveolar and parenchymal disease. Brush specimens are also useful in the diagnosis of bacterial, fungal, mycobacterial, and viral diseases. A sheathed brush protected with a polyethylene glycol plug at the tip is most useful. Topical lidocaine should be kept to a minimum, as it may inhibit bacterial growth.

Special Procedures

1. Transbronchial biopsy is used to evaluate diffuse parenchymal disease, and for local tumors beyond direct endoscopic view. Fluoroscopic guidance of the biopsy forceps, when available, reduces complications, and increases diagnostic yield. Inject a 5 mL bolus of 1:10,000 epinephrine solution into the area to be sampled. Pass the closed forceps out of view and into the involved area. Confirm proper positioning with fluoroscopy. With the forceps passed distally in a small airway, and position confirmed, question the patient regarding chest pain. If pain is present, reposition the forceps. If not, pull the forceps back 2 cm, opened, while the patient inhales, then advance the forceps 2 to 3 cm while the patient exhales. If the patient experiences no pain, close the forceps at the end of expiration and withdraw. Then wedge the tip of the bronchoscope into the bronchial segment for tamponade of any bleeding. If hemorrhage occurs, leave the tip in place for 5 minutes. If no bleeding occurs in 1 minute, remove the bronchoscope and repeat the procedure. Transbronchial biopsies should be performed in one lung only to

prevent the possibility of bilateral pneumothorax. The Wedge technique, introduced in 1976 by Zavala, has significantly decreased the incidence of severe bronchial hemorrhage.

2. The fiberoptic bronchoscope plays a significant role in difficult intubation of patients with facial, upper airway and neck trauma, facial and neck burns, and cervical spine disease such as rheumatoid arthritis.

The degree to which a patient is prepared for the procedure depends on the emergency of the situation. Both oral and nasal intubation can be accomplished. When the oral route is selected, a Williams oral intubator is useful. Prepare the patient and give anesthesia as time permits. Thread an endotracheal tube, 8.5 mm minimum, over the shaft of the lubricated bronchoscope. Insert the bronchoscope into the patient's nose or mouth. Topical anesthesia can be administered through the bronchoscope as time permits. The Williams oral intubator aids in visualization of the epiglottis and vocal cords and serves as a bite block to protect the bronchoscope. Once the tip of the bronchoscope is in the trachea, position it just above the carina. At that point, advance the lubricated endotracheal tube over the shaft of the bronchoscope and into the trachea. Withdraw the bronchoscope, and ventilate the patient with an ambu bag. Subsequently, the endotracheal tube placement can be evaluated bronchoscopically prior to securing the tube in place (see Chapter 18).

3. Bronchoalveolar lavage (BAL) is a useful diagnostic tool in the evaluation of many lung diseases; however, its usefulness in critically ill patients is sometimes limited by an inability to maintain adequate arterial oxygenation. Contraindications to BAL include a forced expiratory volume in 1 second (FEV_1) of less than 1L, a Pao_2 less than 70 mm Hg (with or without supplemental oxygen), acute retention of carbon dioxide (CO_2), unstable cardiovascular disease, and serious electrolyte abnormality. In critically ill patients, BAL is most useful in the evaluation of diffuse lung disease in immunocompromised hosts. Pneumocystis carinii, cytomegalo-

virus, fungi, and acid-fast bacilli can be isolated in BAL fluid. The procedure is not difficult. Wedge a standard adult fiberoptic bronchoscope into a third- or fourth-generation bronchus in the involved area, and inject 20 to 50 mL of sterile normal saline through the working port. Then retrieve the fluid either by gentle suction with the bronchoscope and collection of the fluid in a trap, or by suction with a syringe attached to the working port. A working port syringe is preferred since even gentle wall suction may collapse the airways and decrease the fluid return (especially in patients with emphysema). Total lavage fluid should be 100 mL, with 50% to 75% return. The incidence of complications such as atelectasis, hypoxemia, and transient fever increases when the lavage fluid exceeds 300 mL.

4. Rigid bronchoscopy is the procedure of choice to remove foreign bodies from the central airways, especially in children. However, fiberoptic bronchoscopy can be used to remove small objects from the peripheral airways, which are beyond the reach of the rigid bronchoscope.

Orotracheal intubation is preferred for bronchoscopic removal of a foreign body because it facilitates passage of the foreign body past the glottis and upper airway. A variety of grasping forceps and wire baskets are available to secure an object. When a foreign body cannot be grasped because of interference from surrounding mucosal edema, place a Fogarty catheter beyond the foreign body, inflate, and retract in order to dislodge the foreign body into a larger airway. Complications related to removal of a foreign body include bronchial perforation, displacement of the foreign body to a less favorable location, subglottic airway obstruction, and endobronchial disintegration of the foreign body.

5. When gastric aspiration is suspected as the cause of clinical deterioration or abnormalities are seen on new chest roentgenograms early in the disease condition, fiberoptic bronchoscopy can be useful in establishing the diagnosis. Observation of hemorrhagic tracheo-

bronchitis and mucosal erythema extending into the subsegmental bronchi is suggestive of gastric aspiration, and the finding of gastric contents in the tracheobronchial tree is diagnostic. If large particulate matter is aspirated, rigid bronchoscopy may be necessary.

6. Fiberoptic bronchoscopy is useful in massive pulmonary hemorrhage. If death is threatened because the airways are flooded with blood, use of a rigid bronchoscope is necessary. Otherwise, fiberoptic bronchoscopy is useful in localizing and controlling massive hemoptysis. Localization can be difficult if the airways are loaded with blood, but a fiberoptic bronchoscope is important in subsequent management, which may include bronchial artery embolization or thorocotomy. Control of bleeding can be accomplished with balloon tamponade or with application of epinephrine on a lesion.

7. As part of the burn care team, the bronchoscopist plays a vital role in assessing the integrity of the airway. Heat injury occurs above the vocal cords; the toxic products of combustion cause injury below the vocal cords. Suspect an inhalation in burn patients who have facial and neck burns, singed nasal hair, hoarseness, or carbonaceous material in the nose or sputum.

The most important complication to avoid is obstruction of the airway from an edematous, blistered epiglottis and supraglottic area. When this injury is seen as present on fiberoptic bronchoscopy, immediate intubation is indicated and can be lifesaving.

8. The proper preparation and processing of specimens is essential. Immediately place forceps biopsy material in a container of formalin and send to the pathology department for further histologic processing and examination. Some specimens can be placed in normal saline and sent to the microbiology department for culture and special stains, as indicated.

Washings, which are commonly collected in a trap, should be split, with a portion placed in cytology fixative for subsequent examination and the remainder sent to the microbiology department for special stains and cultures.

Prepare brush specimens by smearing the brush on several glass slides that are properly labeled, and by agitating the brush in a test tube of normal saline. Leave some glass slides to air dry for subsequent acid-fast stain, and immediately place others in fixative or spray with fixative for subsequent Papanicolaou stain.

Special stains that can be done on brushings, washings, and touch preparations of biopsy material include modified acid-fast stain, acid-fast stain, silver methenamine, and legionella immunofluorescence. At our institution, a protocol has been developed for rapid complete processing of specimens from immunocompromised patients.

FOLLOW-UP

Obtaining a follow-up expiratory chest roentgenogram to assess for pneumothorax after transbronchial biopsy is common practice. However, routine chest roentgenograms after transbronchial biospy under fluoroscopic guidance in asymptomatic patients without fluoroscopic evidence of pneumothorax is of low diagnostic yield. A follow-up inspiratory chest roentgenogram to assess the degree of re-expansion of atelectatic lung shows evidence of re-expansion in 85% of patients. Continued monitoring of the heart rate and hemoglobin saturation by oximetry postbronchoscopy is prudent and can aid in assessing the response to therapeutic bronchoscopy.

COMPLICATIONS

Fiberoptic bronchoscopy is generally considered to be a safe procedure; however, it can lead to serious complications. The incidence of serious complications is markedly reduced by careful assessment of risk and adequate precautionary measures. Possible complications are summarized in Table 10–4.

The overall incidence of complications ranges from 8% to 11%, with a mortality rate as high as 0.1% to 0.5% in some prospective studies. Recent retrospective studies report much lower complication rates.

1. Hemorrhage related to biopsy and bushings should be anticipated in patients with a coagulopathy, uremia, immunosuppression, leukemia, bone marrow transplant, vascular tumors, and pulmonary hypertension. Transbronchial biopsy is generally considered too great a risk when one of these conditions exists. Bronchial washings and bronchoalveolar lavage are alternative procedures. In patients without risk factors, significant hemorrhage (defined as more than 50 mL of blood) related to transbronchial biopsy has an incidence of 1%.

2. Pneumothorax is the most common complication of transbronchial biopsy and occurs in 1% to 5.5% of

TABLE 10–4.

Complications of Fiberoptic Bronchoscopy

Adverse reaction to premedication
Adverse reaction to local anesthetic
Vasovagal reaction
Laryngospasm
Bronchospasm
Pneumothorax
Ruptured lung abscess
Hemorrhage
Trauma to the airways
Hypoventilation
Hypoxemia
Cardiac arrhythmia
Myocardial infarction
Postbronchoscopy fever

---

procedures. Death from tension pneumothorax and pulmonary hemorrhage related to transbronchial biopsy has been reported.

3. Flexible fiberoptic bronchoscopy can lead to ventilation-perfusion mismatching and hypoxemia through several mechanisms. An average decrease in Pao_2 of 26% and a mild increase in $Paco_2$ occur in critically ill ventilated patients examined under only midazolam sedation. Risk factors for severe hypoxemia (Pao_2 less than 60 mm Hg on 80% oxygen) include adult respiratory distress syndrome and ineffective ventilation caused by inadequate sedation. A decline in Pao_2 probably occurs to some degree in all ventilated patients undergoing fiberoptic bronchoscopy. Prolonged suctioning has deleterious effects; elimination of PEEP, reduction of lung volume below FRC, and a reduced tidal volume can result. These effects are compounded when short inspiratory times are used with increased airflow resistance. Hypoxemia and hypoventilation may result.

4. A standard therapeutic bronchoscope (outer diameter of 6 mm) inserted into an 8-mm endotracheal tube occupies approximately 50% of its cross-sectional area. The resulting increase in expiratory airflow resistance can cause increased PEEP, which may result in mediastinal emphysema and pneumothorax.

5. Hemodynamic effects include tachycardia, bradycardia, cardiac arrhythmias, increased cardiac output, and increased pulmonary capillary occlusion pressures.

6. Postbronchoscopy infections are uncommon. Temperatures above 101°F orally occur in 15% of procedures, and new pulmonary infiltrates develop in 7%. Serious infections following bronchoscopy include lung abscess, chronic necrotizing pneumonia, gram-negative bacteremia, and septic shock. Evidence to support the use of prophylactic antibiotics in patients at risk for endocarditis is lacking, and prophylaxis is not currently recommended.

Recommendations for reducing the risk of fiberoptic bronchoscopy in critically ill and ventilated patients include the following:

1. Obtain an allergy history.
2. Administer atropine *intramuscularly* prior to the procedure.
3. Manage bronchospasm with inhaled beta agonists, prophylactically if necessary.
4. Manage laryngospasm with inhaled racemic epinephrine.
5. Avoid biopsy and brushing procedures in patients with risk factors for bleeding, or if necessary, attempt to correct the underlying problem prior to the procedure.
6. Use the wedge technique with transbronchial biopsy.
7. Perform transbronchial biopsy with fluoroscopy and in only one lung per procedure.
8. Avoid prolonged suctioning.
9. Increase the fraction of inspired oxygen (F_{IO_2}) to 1.0.
10. Use an endotracheal tube with at least an 8.5-mm inner diameter.
11. Monitor PEEP during the procedure; keep it below 20 cm of water.
12. Use continuous cardiac monitoring.
13. Use continuous pulse oximetry.
14. Obtain a follow-up chest roentgenogram.
15. Use adequate sedation, so the patient does not fight the ventilator.
16. Monitor exhaled tidal volumes.
17. Monitor for adequate chest excursion.

DOCUMENTATION

A preprinted bronchoscopy report, which contains all pertinent information in a concise form, is used at our institution (Fig 10–2). A diagram of the bronchial

FLEXIBLE FIBEROPTIC BRONCHOSCOPY RECORD

INDICATION:

OPERATOR(S):

MEDICATION: Atropine ____ mg;   Demerol ____ mg;   Other _____

ANESTHESIA: Lidocaine ____ ;   Cetacaine ____ ;   Other _____

INSTRUMENT: FLUOROSCOPY: ☐ Yes   ☐ No

APPROACH:

FINDINGS:

    Upper Airway: ____ Normal

    Vocal Cords: ____ Normal

    Trachea: ____ Normal

    Bronchial Tree: ____ Normal

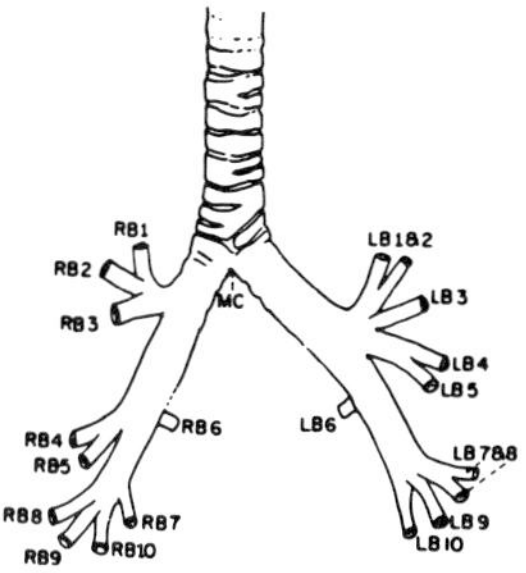

COMPLICATIONS: ____ None

SPECIMENS TAKEN:

    Biopsies: _____   Brushings: _____   Washings: _____

IMPRESSIONS:

RECOMMENDATIONS:

_____ , M.D.   Date: _____

FIG 10–2.
Preprinted bronchoscopy report form. *MC* = main carina; *RB* = right bronchus; *LB* = left bronchus; *RC* = right carina; *LC* = left carina.

anatomy is included on this form to allow us to draw the endobronchial abnormalities encountered. Alternatively, a note in the progress section of the patient's chart can be written and should include:

1. Indication for the procedure
2. Sedation used
3. Evaluation of the preprocedure chest roentgenogram and arterial blood gases analysis
4. Specific findings of the procedure
5. Complications that developed during the procedure

6. Diagnostic specimens taken
7. Postprocedure evaluation of patient's cardiopulmonary function and oxygenation status.

SUGGESTED READING

Bone RC et al: Section report—guidelines for competency and training in fiberoptic bronchoscopy, ACCP guidelines, *Chest* 81:739, 1982.

Credle WF Jr et al: Complications of fiberoptic bronchoscopy, *Am Rev Respir Dis* 109:67–72, 1974.

Dreisin RB et al: Flexible fiberoptic bronchoscopy in the teaching hospital: yield and complications, *Am Rev Respir Dis* 115:102A, 1977.

Ellis JH Jr: Transbronchial lung biopsy via the fiberoptic bronchoscope—experience with 107 consecutive cases and comparison with bronchial brushing, *Chest* 68:524–532, 1975.

Frazier WD, et al: Pneumothorax following transbronchial biopsy—low diagnostic yield with routine chest roentgenograms, *Chest* 97:539–540, 1990.

Herf SM, Suratt PM: Complications of transbronchial lung biopsies, *Chest* 73:759–760, 1978.

Lindholm CE et al: Cardiorespiratory effects of flexible fiberoptic bronchoscopy in critically ill patients, *Chest* 74:362–368, 1978.

Peacock AJ et al: Effect of fiberoptic bronchoscopy on pulmonary function, *Thorax* 45:38–41, 1990.

Pereira W et al: A prospective cooperative study of complications following flexible fiberoptic bronchoscopy, *Chest* 73:813–816, 1978.

Pereira W, et al: Fever and pneumonia after fiberoptic bronchoscopy, *Am Rev Respir Dis* 112:59–64, 1975.

Sokolowski JW Jr et al: Guidelines for fiberoptic bronchoscopy in adults, *Am Rev Respir Dis* 136:1066, 1987.

Suratt PM et al: Deaths and complications associated with fiberoptic bronchoscopy, *Chest* 69:747–751, 1976.

Trouillet JL et al: Fiberoptic bronchoscopy in ventilated patients, *Chest* 97:927–933, 1990.

Wanner A et al: Bedside bronchofiberoscopy for atelectasis and lung abscess, *JAMA* 224:9:1281–1283, 1973.

Wolfe JE et al: Diagnosis of gastric aspiration by fiberoptic bronchoscopy, *Chest* 70:458–459, 1976.

Zavala DC: Bronchoscopy, lung biopsy, and other procedures. In Murray JF, Nadel JA, editors: *Textbook of respiratory medicine*, vol 1, Philadelphia, 1988, WB Saunders.

Zavala DC: Pulmonary hemorrhage in fiberoptic transbronchial biopsy, *Chest* 70:584–588, 1976.

11

Oxygen Therapy

Roy D. Cane, M.B.B.Ch., F.F.A.(S.A.)

INTRODUCTION

Definitions

Hypoxemia is an arterial oxygen partial pressure (Po_2) of less than 80 mm Hg when breathing room air. Hypoxia exists when tissue cellular oxygen tensions are inadequate to maintain aerobic metabolism. Hypoxia may develop because of

1. An inadequate arterial oxygen content (Cao_2) secondary to hypoxemia or anemia
2. Inadequate perfusion
3. Inadequate tissue oxygen uptake or utilization.

Pathophysiology of Tissue Oxygenation

Maintenance of aerobic metabolism depends on a tissue oxygen delivery (Do_2) sufficient to meet tissue oxygen consumption. The product of cardiac output (CO) and arterial oxygen content (Cao_2) reflects the volume of oxygen delivered to the tissues ($Do_2 = CO \times Cao_2$). Reduced Cao_2 secondary to hypoxemia is common in critically ill patients. Hypoxemia may develop by the following mechanisms:

1. Pulmonary disease, which results in
   a. Perfusion of unventilated lung (shunt).
   b. Perfusion greater than ventilation in regions of underventilated lung (shunt effect or venous admixture).
2. Mixed venous blood entering the unventilated lung (shunt) with significantly reduced oxygen content secondary to
   a. Inadequate cardiac output.
   b. Significant anemia without adequate cardiac compensation.
   c. Markedly elevated tissue oxygen consumption without adequate cardiac compensation.

Not all forms of hypoxemia are treated adequately simply by increasing the concentration of inspired oxygen. Underventilation of well-perfused lung units (shunt effect or venous admixture) leads to reduced alveolar oxygen tensions (P_{AO_2}) in these regions of the lung. Blood that passes through a lung unit with a low P_{AO_2} will be incompletely oxygenated; the result is hypoxemia. (See Chapter 9 for a discussion of ventilation-perfusion relationships.) **Hypoxemia as a result of reduced P_{AO_2} secondary to development of ventilation-perfusion mismatching (shunt effect or venous admixture) in the lung is the only type of hypoxemia that responds favorably to oxygen therapy.** Breathing gas mixtures with oxygen concentrations greater than 21%, by increasing P_{AO_2}, may correct hypoxemia. Furthermore, increasing P_{AO_2} may decrease the work of breathing (WOB) required to maintain a given P_{AO_2}. The myocardial work necessary to maintain a given arterial oxygen tension (P_{aO_2}) may also be decreased by breathing gas with a fraction of inspired oxygen (F_{IO_2}) of less than 0.21. Fraction of inspired oxygen is the measurable or calculable concentration of oxygen delivered to the patient.

OBJECTIVE

The goals of oxygen therapy are

1. To correct arterial hypoxemia.
2. To decrease the work of breathing.
3. To decrease the myocardial work.

Indications

1. *Hypoxemia.* Arterial hypoxemia secondary to decreased alveolar oxygen tensions is usually improved by increasing the F_{IO_2}.

2. *Increased work of breathing.* Breathing an oxygen-enriched gas mixture may allow an adequate P_{AO_2} to be maintained with a more normal alveolar minute ventilation, thus decreasing WOB. Furthermore, hypoxemia commonly provokes an increase in ventilation and hence an increase in ventilatory work. Correction of hypoxemia will result in decreased WOB.

3. *Increased myocardial work.* The primary physiologic response to maintain tissue oxygen delivery when hypoxemia develops is an increase in cardiac output. Oxygen therapy that improves arterial oxygenation may result in adequate tissue oxygen delivery with a lower cardiac output, hence, decreasing myocardial work.

Contraindications

None.

PREPARATION

Because excessive concentrations of inspired oxygen are potentially harmful, it is desirable to identify hypoxemic states that are relatively responsive to oxygen therapy. The oxygen challenge, described in Chapter 9, provides a clinical means to identify hypoxemia that is amenable to oxygen therapy. Thus, performance of an oxygen challenge is recommended prior to institution of oxygen therapy.

Equipment

Oxygen therapy may be delivered by rebreathing or non-rebreathing systems. Modern oxygen therapy is properly administered by non-rebreathing systems that deliver either a high or low gas flow.

High-Flow Oxygen Systems

High-flow oxygen systems provide the total inspired atmosphere; the patient breathes only the gas supplied by the apparatus. High-flow systems have two major advantages:

1. Provision of consistent F_{IO_2} irrespective of the patient's ventilatory pattern.
2. Provision of appropriately warmed and humidified inspired gas.

Any oxygen concentration may be administered by high-flow systems. To deliver a given F_{IO_2} consistently, a high-flow system must deliver a fresh gas flow sufficient to meet the patient's minute volume and peak inspiratory flow rate. Adequate flows are achieved by one of two methods:

1. Inclusion of some form of inspiratory reservoir that supplies additional amounts of gas during the transient times when inspiratory flow demands exceed the uniform flow delivered by the apparatus.
2. Provision of an extremely high flow of gas. Although the reservoir of the system is important, the total gas flow rate is undoubtedly the most important

factor. A total gas flow of at least three times the patient's measured minute volume will usually ensure that the peak inspiratory flow demand is met.

Many high-flow oxygen delivery systems use air entrainment to provide a specific F_{IO_2} and gas flow. Air entrainment is achieved by constant-pressure jet mixing, in which the rapid velocity of a gas passing through a restricted orifice creates viscous shearing forces that entrain air into the main gas stream. The air entrainment ratio (and hence F_{IO_2}) depends on orifice and entrainment port size, whereas variation in the oxygen flow rate through the orifice determines the total gas flow delivered by the device. Table 11–1 lists approximate air entrainment ratios for different oxygen concentrations. Values for F_{IO_2} from 0.24 to 0.35 are most frequently provided by air entrainment devices; F_{IO_2} values greater than 0.35 are best provided by systems that deliver adequately high flows of gas with known F_{IO_2}.

Commonly used high-flow oxygen delivery systems include T-piece circuit (Fig 11–1), face mask with wide-bore gas delivery circuit (Fig 11–2), and air entrainment masks (commonly referred to as "venturi masks") (Fig 11–3).

TABLE 11–1.

Approximate Air Entrainment Ratios for Different Oxygen Concentrations*

Oxygen Concentration (%)	Air/oxygen (L/min)
24	25/1
28	10/1
34	5/1
40	3/1
60	1/1
70	0.6/1

*From Oxygen therapy. In Shapiro BA et al: *Clinical application of respiratory care*, ed 4, St Louis, 1991, Mosby–Year Book, p 126. Used by permission.)

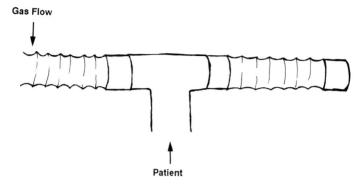

FIG 11–1.
"T" piece circuit; a high-flow gas delivery system suitable for use on intubated patients. Any oxygen concentration can be delivered through this circuit.

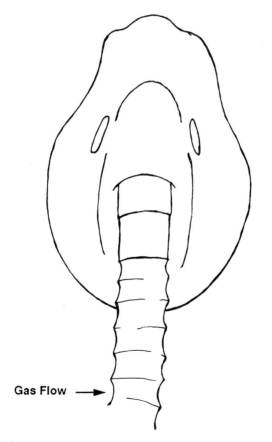

FIG 11–2.
Face mask with wide bore (22 mm) gas delivery tubing; a high-flow gas delivery system for nonintubated patients. Any oxygen concentration can be delivered through this mask.

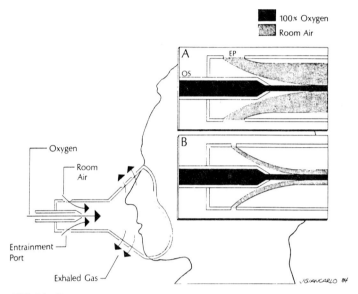

FIG 11–3.
Air entrainment mask. Oxygen flowing at high pressure through the constricted orifice leads to increased gas flow distal to the orifice, which in turn causes air to be entrained through the air entrainment ports. *A* and *B* illustrate how air entrainment ports of different sizes alter the gas mixing, and hence the oxygen concentration. *OS* = oxygen source, *EP* = entrainment port. Because of the limitations of air entrainment, oxygen concentrations greater than 40% can seldom be achieved with a total gas flow that meets requirements for a high-flow gas delivery system. (From Oxygen therapy. In Shapiro BA et al: *Clinical application of respiratory care,* ed 4, St Louis, 1991, Mosby–Year Book, p 127. Used by permission.)

Low-flow Oxygen Systems

Low-flow oxygen systems do not provide sufficient gas flow to supply the entire inspired atmosphere; part of each breath is supplied by breathing room air. A FIO_2 from 0.21 to 0.8 can be provided by a low-flow system. The FIO_2 is determined by

1. The size of the available oxygen reservoir (usually the nose, nasopharynx, and oropharynx)
2. The oxygen flow (L/min)
3. The patient's ventilatory pattern.

In a given patient receiving a preset oxygen flow through a low-flow oxygen delivery system **the F_{IO_2} varies inversely with the minute ventilation.** The larger the tidal volume (V_T), or the faster the respiratory rate, the lower the F_{IO_2}; the smaller the V_T, or the slower the respiratory rate, the higher the F_{IO_2}. Critically ill patients frequently manifest an unstable ventilatory pattern; if delivery of a consistent F_{IO_2} is deemed important, a high-flow system should be used. Commonly used systems for low-flow oxygen delivery include nasal cannula (Fig 11–4), oxygen mask (Fig 11–5), and oxygen mask with reservoir bag (Fig 11–6). Table 11–2 shows approximate F_{IO_2} values that usually will be achieved with these commonly used low-flow oxygen delivery systems provided the patient has a relatively normal ventilatory pattern.

Mouth breathing does not affect the F_{IO_2} delivered by a nasal cannula provided the nasal passages are patent. Airflow in the oropharynx creates a jet mixing effect in the nasopharynx that draws air through the nose. The anatomic reservoir is usually completely filled with oxygen by flows of 6 L/min, thus, further increases in oxygen flow through a nasal cannula seldom result in a higher F_{IO_2}. To provide a higher F_{IO_2} with a low-flow system, the oxygen reservoir has to be increased by placing a mask over the nose and mouth. A potential

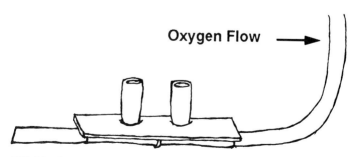

FIG 11–4.
Nasal cannula; a low-flow gas delivery system in which the prongs are placed in the nares. A F_{IO_2} of 0.24 to 0.44 can be delivered with oxygen flows of 1 to 6 L/min.

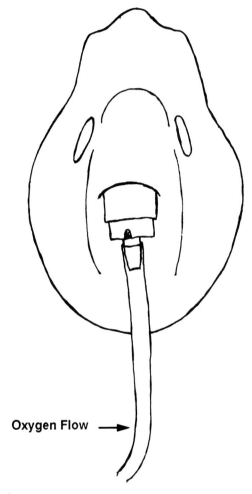

Oxygen Flow ⟶

FIG 11–5.
Simple face mask with small-bore gas delivery tubing. With oxygen flows of 5 to 8 L/min, this mask will deliver an approximate F_{IO_2} of 0.4 to 0.6.

risk with a low-flow face mask is accumulation of exhaled gas in the mask leading to rebreathing. Provision of an oxygen flow greater than 5 L/min will flush most of the exhaled air from the mask. Oxygen flows of 8 L/min will usually fill the mask reservoir, and thus provide the highest F_{IO_2} possible with a low-flow face

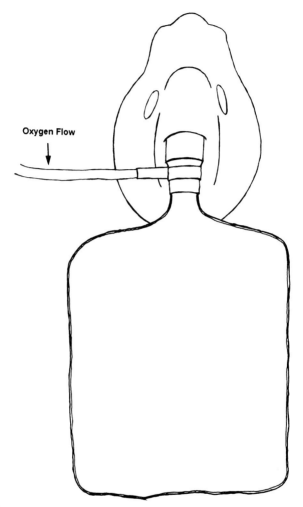

FIG 11–6.
Face mask with addition of a reservoir bag. The addition of the reservoir bag increases the delivered F_{IO_2}. Amounts of F_{IO_2} from 0.6 to over 0.8 are achieved with oxygen flows of 6 to 10 L/min.

mask. To deliver more than 60% oxygen with a low-flow system, the oxygen reservoir has to be further increased by attaching a reservoir bag to the mask. The first one third of the exhaled gas (deadspace gas free of CO_2) will enter the reservoir bag and be breathed again;

TABLE 11–2.

Approximate Fraction of Inspired Oxygen (F_{IO_2}) Values Delivered by Different Low-Flow Oxygen Delivery Systems*†

Nasal Cannula		Oxygen Mask		Mask With Reservoir Bag	
O_2 Flow (L/min)	F_{IO_2}	O_2 Flow (L/min)	F_{IO_2}	O_2 Flow (L/min)	F_{IO_2}
1	0.24	5–6	0.4	6	0.6
2	0.28	6–7	0.5	7	0.7
3	0.32	7–8	0.6	8	0.8
4	0.36	—	—	9	0.8+
5	0.4	—	—	10	0.8+
6	0.44	—	—	—	—

*From Oxygen therapy. In Shapiro BA et al: *Clinical application of respiratory care,* ed 4, Chicago, 1989, Mosby–Year Book, p 129. Used by permission.
†Assumes a normal ventilatory pattern.

thus a mask with reservoir bag is a partial rebreathing system. For proper function, the mask should be close-fitting and the flow of oxygen sufficient to prevent the reservoir bag from totally emptying during inspiration (over 6 L/min).

Required Monitoring

1. Pulse oximetry, though not essential, greatly simplifies oxygen therapy.
2. Vital signs.

Required Laboratory Data

1. Arterial blood gas analysis is desirable. However, in the absence of hypoventilation, pulse oximetry can provide the necessary information.
2. Hemoglobin concentration is desirable. Correction of hypoxemia with oxygen therapy will not ensure adequate arterial oxygenation if the oxygen carrying capacity is impaired as a result of anemia.

PROCEDURE

The following procedure can be employed safely in most patients. Patients with compensated, chronic alveolar hypoventilation (elevated $Paco_2$ with a normal pH) secondary to chronic obstructive pulmonary disease (COPD) require very careful titration of oxygen therapy. (See the following subsection for a discussion of oxygen therapy for COPD patients.)

1. Establish the presence of hypoxemia by measurement of Pao_2 or pulse oximetry.
2. Consider performing an oxygen challenge (see Chapter 9) to determine whether the hypoxemia will respond to breathing gas with augmented oxygen concentrations. Although this step is not essential, if the patient's condition and time permit, it provides useful information regarding choice of Fio_2.
3. Establish baseline vital signs. Improvement in heart rate and respiratory rate, and reduction in systolic hypertension, are clinical indicators of adequate oxygen therapy.
4. Measure the patient's minute volume.
5. Select an oxygen delivery system. A high-flow system is recommended if any of the following pertain.
   a. The patient has an unstable breathing pattern.
   b. Hypoxemia is severe ($Pao_2 < 55$ mm Hg or arterial oxygen saturation Spo_2 under 85%), necessitating a Fio_2 greater than 0.35.
   c. The patient has a measured minute volume more than 6 to 7 L.
   d. The patient is intubated (high-flow systems allow for provision of appropriately humidified gas).
      Air entrainment devices are reliable for delivery of Fio_2 up to 0.35. At higher Fio_2 an air entrainment device may not deliver a gas flow sufficient to meet the patient's minute volume and peak inspiratory

flow demands. If an air entrainment device is used for a F_{IO_2} greater than 0.35, measure the gas flow delivered by the system to ensure that it exceeds three times the patient's measured minute volume.

Low-flow oxygen delivery systems are usually reliable for patients with relatively normal minute ventilation and stable breathing patterns. The specific low-flow device selected will in part depend on the desired F_{IO_2} (see Table 11–2). Frequently the breathing pattern will stabilize once an adequate F_{IO_2} is provided, thus allowing for a switch to a more comfortable, less expensive low-flow system after the patient has been stabilized.

6. Select the desired F_{IO_2}. In an emergency situation always place the patient on an F_{IO_2} of 1.0. In nonemergency circumstances, start with a F_{IO_2} of 0.4 to 0.5; adequate correction of hypoxemia due to shunt effect or venous admixture usually is obtained with F_{IO_2} of 0.5 or less. Inadequate Pao_2 or arterial saturation, as measured with pulse oximetry (Spo_2), on a F_{IO_2} of 0.5, usually reflects that the hypoxemia is predominantly as a result of mechanisms other than shunt effect or venous admixture.

7. Evaluate the patient's response to oxygen therapy. Measure Spo_2 or Pao_2. A Spo_2 between 92% to 95% or Pao_2 between 80 to 100 mm Hg are classic endpoints for oxygen therapy. Given that the Cao_2 is not significantly further increased by an Spo_2 greater than 90% or Pao_2 greater than 60 mm Hg, many clinicians will accept these values as endpoints to enable use of the lowest possible F_{IO_2}. Improvement in vital signs is a reliable sign that adequate arterial oxygenation has been achieved.

8. Titrate the F_{IO_2} to the lowest value that maintains adequate arterial oxygenation. Pulse oximetry provides the simplest and safest means of titrating the F_{IO_2}.

Oxygen Therapy for Patients With COPD and Chronic Alveolar Hypoventilation

Patients with COPD who have chronic elevation of $Paco_2$ **may** hypoventilate in response to arterial hyperoxia. The mechanism of hyperoxia-induced hypoventilation is not understood. Whatever the mechanism, for practical clinical purposes it is wise to assume that these patients will behave as though they depend on a hypoxic ventilatory drive, and to modify the approach to delivery of oxygen therapy accordingly.

1. Establish the presence of acute hypoxemia. Remember that a COPD patient usually will have a markedly reduced Pao_2 (usually less than 60 mm Hg) when they are well. Suspect acute hypoxemia if examination of the patient reveals acute respiratory distress. In the early phase of an acute cardiopulmonary problem these patients often will hyperventilate and arterial blood gases (ABG) analysis will show an acute alveolar hyperventilation superimposed on chronic alveolar hypoventilation ($Paco_2$ elevated, with pHa greater than 7.40). Careful monitoring of respiratory rate, heart rate, and subjective feelings of ease/difficulty of breathing provide the best indicators of the oxygenation status of the patient.

2. **Do not perform an oxygen challenge.** Hypoxemia secondary to COPD is usually due to shunt effect/venous admixture and is very responsive to increases in the Fio_2.

3. Select an oxygen delivery system. Low-flow delivery systems are not recommended for initiation of oxygen therapy in COPD patients with unstable cardiopulmonary function. Because the Fio_2 delivered by a low-flow system varies inversely with the minute ventilation, any inadvertent hyperoxia that results in hypoventilation will lead to an increase in Fio_2 that, in turn, will result in further hypoventilation. Thus, a vicious cycle can be established that will ultimately result in acute ventilatory failure. A high-flow system

that delivers a consistent F_{IO_2} independent of changes in the patient's breathing pattern and minute ventilation provides the safest method for delivery of oxygen therapy for the COPD patient. As these patients seldom require high F_{IO_2}s or have large minute volumes, air entrainment masks are reliable systems.

4. Select the F_{IO_2}. Start with an F_{IO_2} of 0.24 and evaluate the patient's response to oxygen therapy.

5. Titrate the F_{IO_2} in increments of 0.04 to 0.05. The desirable endpoint of oxygen therapy is best determined by demonstration of normalization of the respiratory rate, heart rate, and arterial pH (pHa). The patient will usually state that his/her breathing feels easier when appropriate arterial oxygenation has been restored. The actual value of Pao_2 or Spo_2 will depend on the degree of underlying COPD and, invariably, will be less than 60 mm Hg or 90%. Prior knowledge of the patient's usual ABG values is of considerable benefit in determining the endpoint of oxygen therapy. It is essential to check that the patient maintains adequate ventilation. Values for ABG reflecting a pHa of 7.35 to 7.4 in conjunction with stable vital signs are reassuring.

6. Once the patient's condition has stabilized and the appropriate therapy for the underlying acute disease process instituted, it is reasonable to use a low-flow system (nasal cannula) to enhance patient comfort. Remember that the guidelines for delivered F_{IO_2} outlined in Table 11−2 are based on a normal minute volume and, therefore, will probably overestimate the F_{IO_2} that will be achieved in the COPD patient. Therefore, titrate the oxygen flow rate through the nasal cannula to the endpoints discussed earlier.

FOLLOW-UP

1. Maintain surveillance of the adequacy of arterial oxygenation. Continuous pulse oximetry is best. If pulse oximetry is unavailable or is precluded by specific patient factors (such as lack of sites for application of the

sensor, or very poor peripheral perfusion), intermittent ABG analysis should be done. The frequency of ABG analysis will depend on the stability of the patient's condition. Frequent ABG sampling is best achieved by placement of an indwelling arterial catheter (see Chapter 1). Transcutaneous Po_2 ($Ptco_2$) monitoring is an alternative noninvasive technique for monitoring the oxygenation status. However, $Ptco_2$ monitoring is less reliable than pulse oximetry, depends on blood flow to the skin, and probably should be used only as a trend monitor.

2. When the patient's condition improves, reduce the Fio_2 in 0.05 to 0.1 decrements. Provide the minimal Fio_2 that maintains adequate arterial oxygenation.

3. For patient comfort, consider use of a low-flow system once the patient manifests a stable breathing pattern and does not require an Fio_2 of over 0.35.

COMPLICATIONS

1. *Denitrogenation absorption atelectasis.* Nitrogen, a physiologically inert gas, freely distributes throughout the body, and nitrogen tensions (Pn_2) are nearly equal in the alveolar gas and blood under steady-state conditions. Presence of significant volumes of nitrogen in the alveoli help to stabilize the alveoli by keeping them above a critical volume. Administration of 100% oxygen will result in elimination of nitrogen from the body within 15 minutes. Figure 11–7 is a schematic representation of how denitrogenation of well perfused but underventilated alveoli may result in decreasing alveolar volume. If the alveolar volume falls below a critical value, the alveolus will collapse, creating a perfused, nonventilated unit (shunt). Thus, denitrogenation, by creating shunt units, may lead to worsening hypoxemia. Clinically significant denitrogenation absorption atelectasis can develop on Fio_2s greater than 0.5.

2. *Oxygen toxicity.* Cellular metabolism of oxygen involves sequential reduction of oxygen to water and gen-

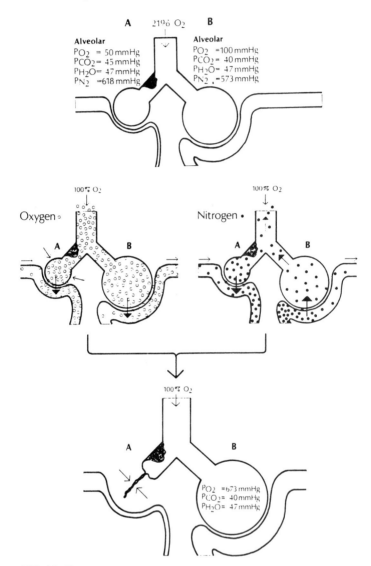

FIG 11–7.
Diagrammatic representation of the mechanism of denitrogenation absorption atelectasis. Alveolus *A* has low V/Q relationships (minimal ventilation), alveolus *B* has normal V/Q relationships. The *top panel* shows the alveolar partial pressures when breathing room air. The *center panel* shows the effect of breathing 100% oxygen. The high F_{IO_2} results in loss of hypoxic

erates so-called oxygen free radicals (superoxide molecule and a hydroxyl ion) during the process. These oxygen free radicals are metabolically highly reactive and have the potential to disrupt cellular function. Normal lung contains enzyme systems (superoxide dismutase is the best characterized) that regulate and control these free radicals. Exposure to F_{IO_2} of over 0.6 for periods greater than 72 to 96 hours may result in pulmonary cellular damage and development of a clinical picture consistent with acute lung injury. It is believed that this lung damage results from the generation of large amounts of oxygen free radicals that overwhelm the lung's regulatory capacity. This circumstance has been termed oxygen toxicity. As prolonged exposure to a F_{IO_2} greater than 0.6 is necessary for the development of oxygen toxicity, it is an uncommon problem if the principles of oxygen therapy outlined in this chapter are followed. Because the possibility exists that non-oxygen-induced lung disease may result in a diminished capacity of the lung to control and regulate the development of oxygen free radicals, many clinicians believe that the lowest possible F_{IO_2} that results in adequate arterial oxygenation should be used at all times.

---

pulmonary vasoconstriction, and blood flow to alveolus *A* increases. The increased blood flow to this poorly ventilated alveolus results in significantly increased oxygen extraction, which in turn results in a diminished gas volume in alveolus *A*. *Black circles* represent nitrogen, which is rapidly depleted from all units secondary to the fact that inspired nitrogen concentration is now zero. Initially, more nitrogen leaves the blood and the body by way of unit *B* because it is better ventilated. As the blood P_{N_2} level progressively decreases, however, nitrogen will start to leave alveolus *A* through the blood. This results in further loss of gas volume from alveolus *A* because it remains poorly ventilated but well perfused. Thus, nitrogen is depleted from all units within 5 to 15 minutes. The *bottom panel* represents a final steady state in which increased oxygen and nitrogen extraction has caused alveolus *A* to collapse. Thus, a poorly ventilated, poorly perfused unit *A* becomes a nonventilated, poorly perfused unit after administration of 100% inspired oxygen. (From Limitations of oxygen therapy. In Shapiro BA et al: *Clinical application of respiratory care*, ed 4, St Louis, 1991, Mosby–Year Book, p 144. Used by permission.)

DOCUMENTATION

Write orders for oxygen therapy that include the following.

1. Oxygen delivery system.
2. The F_{IO_2}.
3. Monitoring (either A or B).
   a. Continuous pulse oximetry.
   b. Frequency of ABG analysis.
4. High and low limits for either Sp_{O_2} or Pa_{O_2} which, if exceeded, necessitate notification of the responsible physician.

SUGGESTED READING

Shapiro BA et al: Hypoxemia and oxygen therapy. In *Clinical application of blood gases*, ed 4, St Louis 1989. Mosby–Year Book.

Shapiro BA et al: Oxygen therapy. In *Clinical application of respiratory care*, ed 4, St Louis, 1991, Mosby–Year Book.

12

Bronchial Hygiene Therapy

Roy D. Cane, M.B.B.Ch., F.F.A.(S.A.)

INTRODUCTION

Spontaneous bronchial hygiene involves two primary mechanisms: the mucociliary escalator and the cough mechanism.

Mucociliary Escalator

The ciliated epithelium of the tracheobronchial tree is completely covered by a mucus blanket comprised of a superficial gel layer and a deep sol layer. The ciliary action moves the mucus blanket in a continuous cephalad direction to the pharynx, where the mucus is swallowed. The mucociliary escalator mechanism is illustrated in Figure 12–1. This process of mucokinesis depends on appropriate ciliary action and normal mucus production.

Ciliary action is depressed by smoking, foreign bodies in the trachea (for example, an endotracheal tube),

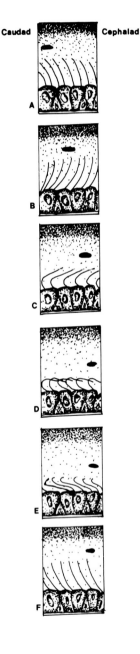

positive pressure ventilation, high inspired oxygen concentrations, tracheobronchial disease, dehydration, and general anesthesia.

Cough Mechanism

An effective cough requires a deep inspiration, end inspiratory pause, exhalation against a closed glottis until airway pressure rises, and an explosive expiratory gas flow when the glottis opens (Figure 12–2). The couch mechanism is initiated by stimulation of vagal afferents by a foreign body in, or irritation of, the tracheobronchial tree. The high-velocity exhalation of a cough mobilizes mucus; the more fluid the mucus and the more complete the mucus blanket, the more effective will be the cough. The cough mechanism, when the mucociliary escalator fails to maintain normal bronchial hygiene, becomes the major pulmonary defense against retention of tracheobronchial secretions. Circumstances that result in an impaired cough mechanism are listed in Table 12–1.

Inadequate bronchial hygiene leads to retention of secretions, which in turn has the potential to disrupt normal lung function. In Figure 12–3 the potential consequences of retained secretions are demonstrated.

The term "bronchial hygiene therapy" (BHT) de-

←FIG 12–1.

The mucociliary escalator consists of the ciliated epithelium covered by a blanket of mucus which has a luminal gel layer and a sol layer between the gel layer and the ciliated surface of the cells lining the trachea. *A* shows the cilia extended with their tips in the gel layer. *B* and *C* show the cilia wafting in a cephalad direction, which serves to drag the gel layer of mucus cephalad over the sol layer; note that the *black spot* moves cephalad. *D* shows the cilia retracting so that their tips leave the gel layer and lie in the sol layer of mucus. *E* shows the retracted cilia wafting in a caudad direction; note that because the tips of the cilia are in the sol layer they do *not* drag the gel layer back and the *black spot* remains on the cephalad side of the figure. *F* shows the cilia extending into the gel layer prior to starting the cycle again. This process keeps the gel layer of mucus moving in a cephalad direction.

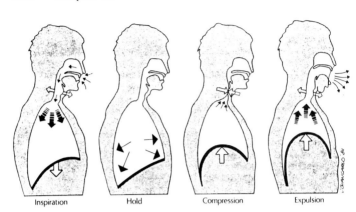

| Inspiration | Hold | Compression | Expulsion |

FIG 12–2.
Diagrammatic representation of a cough. *Inspiration* reflects a deep breath. *Hold* depicts an end inspiratory pause during which optimal peripheral distribution of ventilation is achieved. *Compression* depicts exhalation against a closed glottis with resultant increasing airway pressure. *Expulsion* shows opening of the glottis and forceful exhalation. (From Retained secretions. In Shapiro BA et al: *Clinical application of respiratory care*, ed 4, Chicago, 1991, Mosby–Year Book, p 52. Used by permission.)

scribes various modalities of respiratory care that are employed to augment inadequate spontaneous bronchial hygiene. The goals of BHT are listed in Table 12–2. Aerosol therapy is delivered with either pneumatic or ultrasonic nebulizers. Intermittent positive pressure therapy includes intermittent positive pressure breathing (IPPB), ambu and inflation hold, and in-

TABLE 12–1.

Factors Associated With Impaired Cough Mechanism

Inadequate inspiratory capacity (IC)
  IC < 75% normal
  Vital capacity < 15 mL/kg
Inadequate inspiratory pause
  Rapid respiratory rate
Inability to close glottis
  Intubation
  Glottic paralysis
Inability to increase airway pressure
  Poor or absent expiratory muscle
    function

Potential Results of Retained Secretions

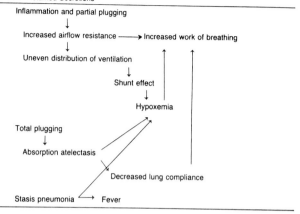

FIG 12–3.
Schematic representation of potential results of retention of pulmonary secretions. (From Shapiro BA et al: Retained secretions. In *Clinical application of respiratory care*, ed 4, St Louis, Mosby–Year Book, 1991. Used by permission.)

termittent mask continuous positive airway pressure (CPAP). Chest physical therapy (CPT) includes postural drainage, chest wall percussion, and vibration. Sustained maximal inspiration therapy (SMI) involves use of devices (incentive spirometers) that encourage a sustained, slow inspiration. The modality of choice for prophylactic BHT in patients with changes in lung function that predispose to reduced cough efficacy, retained secretions, and atelectasis is SMI.

OBJECTIVE

Mobilization of retained tracheobronchial secretions and reversal of pulmonary pathophysiologic consequences of retained secretions.

Indications

1. Retained secretions.
2. Atelectasis.
3. Poor spontaneous cough.

TABLE 12–2.

Goals of Bronchial Hygiene Therapy

Goals of aerosol therapy
    Aid bronchial hygiene
        Restore and maintain mucous blanket continuity
        Hydrate dried, retained secretions
        Promote expectoration
    Humidify inspired gases
    Deliver medication
Goals of intermittent positive pressure breathing therapy
    Improve and promote cough mechanism
    Improve distribution of ventilation
    Deliver medication
Goals of chest physical therapy
    Aid bronchial hygiene
        Prevent accumulation of bronchial secretions
        Promote mobilization of bronchial secretions
        Improve the cough mechanism
    Improve efficiency and distribution of ventilation
Goals of sustained maximal inspiration therapy
    Optimize lung inflation
        Prevent atelectasis
        Prevent accumulation of bronchial secretions
    Optimize cough mechanism
    Enable early detection of acute pulmonary disease

Contraindications

Absolute: None.

Relative: Unstable cardiac function.

Certain modalities of BHT may be contraindicated in specific clinical circumstances because of limitations on patient positioning. For example, the head-down or supine position may not be tolerated by patients with intracranial hypertension or cardiac failure.

PREPARATION

Equipment

Depending on the particular modality of BHT to be used, the following may be necessary:

1. Incentive spirometer.
2. Suction apparatus.
3. Self-inflating manual ventilator (for example, ambu bag).
4. IPPB machine.
5. Free-flowing CPAP circuit with face mask.

Required Monitoring

1. Continuous electrocardiography.
2. Pulse oximetry.

Required Laboratory Data

A chest roentgenogram, although not required, is desirable to facilitate diagnosis of underlying indication for, and response to, BHT.

PROCEDURE

1. Determine the underlying bronchial hygiene problem, such as poor cough, retained secretions, and/or atelectasis.
2. Evaluate spontaneous bronchial hygiene capability by
   a. Measurement of inspiratory capacity or vital capacity.
   b. Observation of spontaneous cough.
   c. Examination of viscosity of sputum.
3. Select the modalities of BHT to be used. Table 12–3 is a list of the various modalities, their actions, and specific indications. These modalities are frequently used in combinations. (Table 12–4).
4. Formulate a plan of BHT including modalities to be used, frequency of therapy, and duration of therapy. Patients with respiratory distress secondary to retained secretions or atelectasis should receive BHT every 4 hours; therapy four times daily when

TABLE 12–3.

Indications for and Effects of Bronchial Hygiene Therapy (BHT) Regimes*†

BHT Modality	Effect	Indications
Ultrasonic nebulization of 0.5N saline	Liquefies inspissated mucus	Thick, retained secretions
Aerosolized beta agonist	Enhances mucociliary transport; bronchodilatation	Retained secretions
Aerosolized mucolytic	Liquefies inspissated mucus	Retained secretions
Chest physical therapy		
Postural drainage	Mobilizes mucus	Thin, retained secretions
Percussion and vibration	Loosens and mobilizes mucus; re-expands collapsed lung	Retained secretions; atelectasis
IPPB in a cooperative, nonintubated patient	Augments inspiratory capacity and improves cough	Poor cough with VC < 15 mL/kg
Ambu and inflation hold, intubated patient	Mimics spontaneous cough	Retained secretions; atelectasis
Intermittent mask CPAP	Augments FRC; re-expands collapsed lung	Poor cough with low VC; atelectasis
SMI (incentive spirometry)	Augments basilar lung ventilation	Prophylaxis and treatment of retained secretions and atelectasis

*From Retained secretions. In Shapiro BA et al: *Clinical application of respiratory care,* ed 4, St Louis, 1991, Mosby–Year Book, p 53. Used by permission.
†IPPB = Intermittent positive pressure breathing; VC = vital capacity; CPAP = continuous positive airway pressure; FRC = functional residual capacity; SMI = sustained maximal inspiration therapy.

the patient is awake, is sufficient for patients not in respiratory distress.

FOLLOW-UP

After 24 hours of bronchial hygiene therapy, the following should be performed.

1. Review respiratory therapist's notes to determine
   a. Whether the treatments produced secretions, and the volume and nature of those secretions.

TABLE 12–4.

Bronchial Hygiene Regimen*†

Findings	Therapy
Inspissated secretions with or without wheezing	
Retained—adequate vital capacity (VC)	USN/CPT + beta agonist
Retained—inadequate VC	IPPB/USN (± CPT) + beta agonist
Able to mobilize secretions	USN ± beta agonist
Loose secretions with wheezing	Aerosol beta agonist ± CPT
Wheezing without secretions	Aerosol beta agonist
Atelectasis	USN/CPT (± beta agonist)
Benefit-of-doubt	
Postoperative fever	USN + IS
Chronic lung disease with questionable acute symptoms or findings	USN + beta agonist
No identifiable bronchial hygiene problem	
Postoperative	IS
Bedridden	IS

*From Applying and evaluating bronchial hygiene therapy: In Shapiro BA et al: In *Clinical application of respiratory care*, ed 4, St Louis, 1991, Mosby–Year Book, p 86. Used by permission.
†USN = ultrasonic nebulizer; CPT = chest physical therapy; IPPB = intermittent positive pressure breathing; IS = inspirometer.

    b. Whether the patient developed significant arterial hypoxemia or arrhythmias during BHT.
2. Examine the patient, evaluate the post-BHT chest roentgenogram, and adjust modalities and frequency as needed.

COMPLICATIONS

Despite a number of anecdotal case reports, little prospective documentation of significant complications of BHT exists. Clinical experience suggest that BHT is not associated with significant complications. Complications encountered are attributable to the following: the side effects of medications used in conjunction with aerosol treatments; disruption of the fraction of inspired oxygen (F$_{IO_2}$); endotracheal suctioning; and application of positive airway pressure.

1. Hypoxemia of mild degree is commonly encountered during and for several minutes after endotracheal suctioning and CPT.
2. Cardiac arrhythmias may occur, particularly during endotracheal suctioning and CPT.
3. Complications associated with mechanical lung inflation by IPPB include the following.
   a. Increased airway resistance. Bronchospasm, especially in asthmatics, may be precipitated by IPPB.
   b. Although not common, barotrauma in association with IPPB has been documented. Once again, this problem occurs more frequently in asthmatic patients.
   c. Nosocomial pneumonia. The reservoir nebulizer, use of multi-dose bottles for aerosolized medications, and the IPPB circuit have all been implicated as sources of nosocomial infection.
   d. Miscellaneous conditions. Gastric distention, hyperventilation, impedance of venous return, and impaction of secretions are frequently listed as complications of IPPB; however, no reliable documentation exists regarding these complications.
4. Complications of intermittent CPAP. Although continuous application of CPAP is associated with well-described complications, no undesirable effects associated with the intermittent application of low levels of CPAP by face mask have been reported.

DOCUMENTATION

Describe the evaluation of the patient's spontaneous bronchial hygiene capabilities, and provide the rationale for the choice of BHT modalities and frequency of treatments.

SUGGESTED READING

Shapiro BA et al: Bronchial hygiene therapy. In *Clinical application of respiratory care,* ed 4; St Louis, 1991, Mosby–Year Book, pp 49–108.

Shapiro BA et al: Complications of mechanical aids to intermittent lung inflation, *Respir Care* 27:467–70, 1982.

13

Sedation and Pain Management in the Critically Ill

Joan M. Christie, M.D.
Susan Markowsky, Pharm. D.

INTRODUCTION

Pain in the Intensive Care Unit (ICU) patient commonly is undertreated, often because of fears of narcotic-induced ventilatory depression or cardiovascular instability. Assessing pain and evaluating analgesic outcome are very difficult in the critically ill, compounding the challenges of pain management in this setting.

Postoperative pain continues to be a substantive problem for both patients and physicians. Despite recent advances in treatment options, the prevalence of acute postoperative pain has remained unchanged for 30 years. The need for analgesia in the intensive care unit is unequivocal, impacting on such disparate phenomena as pulmonary morbidity and length of hospital stay. While newer analgesic technologies have become ubiquitous in the operating room, they are not always

154

found in the ICU. Clearly the ineffectiveness of analgesia in the ICU is due more to the manner in which analgesics are utilized than to the specific nature of the analgesics themselves.

Opiates, sedative hypnotics, and major tranquilizers commonly are prescribed for the critically ill and represent an important component of many aspects of intensive care. This chapter deals with the use of narcotic analgesics, benzodiazepines, and phenothiazine derivatives in the ICU for the treatment of pain, anxiety, and psychosis.

OBJECTIVE

To define the use and routes of administration of opiates, benzodiazepines, and major tranquilizers in the treatment of pain, anxiety, and psychosis in the ICU.

Opiate analgesics (Table 13-1)

Indications

1. To provide analgesia after surgery or trauma.
2. To provide analgesia for procedures such as wound care or line placement.
3. To augment the sedative effects of anxiolytic or antipsychotic medications.
4. To treat symptomatic opiate withdrawal.

Contraindications

1. Restlessness, hypertension, or tachycardia secondary to metabolic effects such as hypoglycemia, hypoxia, hypercarbia, sepsis, or concomitant drug administration.
2. Raised intracranial pressure.
3. Untreated closed-angle glaucoma.
4. Allergies to the specific narcotic.

TABLE 13–1.

Narcotic Analgesics

Drug	Route*	Onset (hr)	Half-life (hr)	Dosing Interval	EAD† (mg)	Active Metabolites
Codeine	IM/IV	0.5–1	2–4	q 3–4 hr	130	Morphine
	PO	0.5–1		q 3–4 hr	200	
Hydromorphone	IM/IV	0.25–0.5	2–3	q 4 hr	1.5	None
	PO	0.5		q 4 hr	7.5	
Levorphanol	IV/SC	0.5–1.5	12–16	q 5–6 hr	2	None
	PO	1		q 4–6 hr	4	
Meperidine	IM/IV	0.5	2–4	q 3–4 hr	75–100	Normeperidine§ (half-life, 8–21 hr)
	PO	0.5–1.5		q 4–5 hr	300	
Methadone	IM/IV	0.33	≥ 24	q 6–8 hr	10	None
	PO	0.5–1		q 6–8 hr‡	10–20	
Morphine	IM/IV	0.5–1	2–5	q 3–4 hr	10	Morphine-6-Glucuronide
	PO	0.5–1.5		q 3–4 hr	30–60	Morphine-3-Glucuronide
	SR PO	1.5–3		q 8–12 hr	30	
	SC continuous	0.5–1		2–10 mg/h	10	
	Epidural—single dose	1.5–2		12–24 hr	1.5–5	
	Epidural—continuous	1.5–2		Continuous infusion	.25–1mg/hr	
Oxycodone	PO	0.5	2–4	q 4–6 hr	15	Oxymorphone
Propoxyphene	PO	0.5–1	6–12	q 3–4 hr	500	Norpropoxyphene§ (half-life 30–36 hr)

*IM = intramuscular; IV = intravenous; PO = by mouth; SR = sustained release; SC = subcutaneous.
†EAD = Equivalent analgesic doses: all doses listed have equivalent analgesic potency to 10 mg of intramuscular morphine sulfate.
‡Duration of action increases to 8 to 48 hours with repeated oral administration.
§Active metabolites may accumulate in patients with renal failure.

Benzodiazepines (Table 13-2)

Indications

1. For preoperative sedation.
2. To provide conscious sedation before short diagnostic or therapeutic procedures such as bronchoscopy, gastroscopy, or wound debridement.
3. To provide short-term relief of symptoms of anxiety.
4. For the treatment of delirium tremens associated with acute alcoholic withdrawal.
5. To treat skeletal muscle spasm.

Contraindications

1. Known hypersensitivity to benzodiazepines.
2. Acute untreated narrow-angle glaucoma.
3. Pregnancy. Teratogenicity has occurred.
4. Psychotic episodes will not respond to benzodiazepines.
5. Endogenous depression will not respond and may worsen with benzodiazepines.

Phenothiazines and Buterophenones (Table 13−3)

Indications

1. For the management of manifestations of psychotic disorders.
2. For control of ticks and vocal utterances in patients with Tourette's disorder.
3. For acute delerium unassociated with hypoxia, hypoglycemia, or other metabolic disorders.

Contraindications

1. Parkinsons disease.
2. Hypersensitivity.
3. Toxic central nervous system depression.

TABLE 13-2.
Benzodiazepines/Anxiolytics

Drug	Route*	Onset	Half-life (t-½) (hr)	Dosing Interval	Dose (mg)	Active Metabolites (t-½, hr)
Alprazolam	PO	Intermediate	11-15	q 8 hr	0.25-0.5	Alpha-Hydroxyalprazolam
Chlordiazepoxide	PO IV/IM†	Intermediate	5-30	q 4-6 hr	5-25	Demoxepam (14-95) Desmethylchlor-Diazepoxide (18) Desmethyldiazepam (36-200) Oxazepam (3-21)
Clorazepate	PO	Rapid	Pro-drug‡ 2.0	q 4-8 hr	3.75-15	Desmethyldiazepam (36-200) Oxazepam (3-21)
Diazepam	PO IV/IM†	Rapid	20-50	q 6-8 hr q 2-4 hr	2-10 2-10	Desmethyldiazepam (36-200) Oxazepam (3-21)

Drug	Route*	Onset	Half-life (hr)	Dose (mg)	Dosing interval	Active metabolite (half-life, hr)
Flurazepam	PO	Intermediate	Pro-drug‡ 1.3	15–30	qhs	Desalkylflhiraepam (50-100)
Lorazepam	PO IV/IM	Rapid	10–20	0.5–4 0.5–4	q 8 hr	None
Midazolam	IV/IM†	Rapid	2–3 1–20§	0.5–2 0.5–6mg/hr	q 4–8 hr q 1–2 hr‖ Continuous infusion	Alpha-Hydroxymidazolam (1-1.3)
Oxazepam	PO	Slow to intermediate	5–10	10–30	q 6–8 hr	None
Prazepam	PO	Slow	Pro-drug‡ 1.3	5–10 20	q 6–8 hr qhs	Desmethyldiazepam (36-200) Oxazepam (3-21)

*PO = by mouth; IV = intravenous; IM = intramuscular.
†Parent drug and active metabolite may accumulate and have a prolonged effect with repeated dosing.
‡See active metabolite column.
§Half-lives reported for intensive care patients vary widely.
‖Continuous infusion rate following 1-mg loading dose.

TABLE 13–3.
Profile of Major Phenothiazines and Related Antipsychotics

Drug	Route*	Onset (hr)	Half-life (hr)	Dosing Interval	Dose (mg)	Active Metabolites	Alpha Blockade†	EPS‡
Chlorpromazine	PO	0.5–1.0	20–40	q 4–6 hr	10–25	7-Hydroxy-chlorpromazine	++ +	++
	IV	0.5		q 4–6 hr	12.5–50			
Haloperidol	PO	0.5	12–36	q 4–6 hr	2–4	Reduced haloperidol	+	+++
	IV			q 3–6 hr	1–5			
Proclorperazine	PO	0.5	10–24	q 6–8 hr	5–10	None	+	++
	IV§	0.5		q 4–6 hr	2.5–10			
Thioridazine	PO	0.5	9–30	q 4–6 hr	25–100	Mesoridazine sulphoridazine	++	+

*PO = by mouth; IV = intravenous.
†++ += ; ++ =.
‡Extrapyramidal side effects.
§Not recommended subcutaneously secondary to local irritation.

4. Patients who have previously experienced tardive dyskinesia.

5. Patients who have previously experienced neuroleptic malignant syndrome.

6. Hypotension. Phenothiazines are alpha-blockers and may continue to lower the blood pressure.

7. Patients receiving anticonvulsive medications or patients with a seizure history. Phenothiazines may lower convulsive threshold.

Routes of Administration

The benzodiazepines and phenothiazines may be given by intravenous (IV) or intramuscular (IM) routes, or orally (see Tables 13-2 and 13-3.)

Opiates may be administered intravenously, subcutaneously, by mouth, via the intrathecal route, or by means of an epidural catheter. This section will outline some considerations for the various routes of administration available for opiate analgesics.

1. Patients with functional gastrointestinal systems who will be discharged soon from the ICU could receive analgesics by mouth.

2. Many patients in the ICU will receive their opiates through the IV route. Agents can be titrated easily to the desired endpoint either by a nurse or by the patient using a patient-controlled analgesia (PCA) device. The PCA method is preferred for cognizant patients who are hemodynamically stable (Table 13-4).

3. Intramuscular injections increase patient discomfort and may engender skin breakdown in immobilized ICU patients. Intramuscular injections interfer with some important tests, such as creatinine phosphokinase, and are rarely indicated in the ICU.

4. Continuous subcutaneous infusion remains an acceptable option for burned patients or patients for whom IV access is otherwise difficult. Loading doses and volume of infusion are particularly important for subcuta-

TABLE 13-4.

Patient-Controlled Analgesia

Opiate Preparation	Loading Dose (mg)	Basal Rate (mL)	Lockout Interval (min)	Demand Dose (mL)
Hydromorphine 0.2 mg/mL	0.2	0-1.5	6-10	0.5-2
Meperidine 10 mg/mL	10	None*	6-10	0.5-2
Morphine 1 mg/mL	1-4	0-2	6-10	0.5-2

*Normeperidine, an active metabolite, may accumulate.

neous infusions during development of steady-state kinetics (see Table 13-1).

5. An epidural technique is preferred for patients who will benefit from very small doses of opiate, for example, head-injured patients with pain who may develop increased intracranial pressure or clouded sensorium with systemic opiates. The epidural route is indicated after chest trauma and for major abdominal procedures, to decrease splinting and help prevent postoperative pulmonary complications. Epidural catheters are contraindicated when patients are receiving anticoagulants, have infection at the proposed catheter insertion site, or refuse the procedure.

PREPARATION

Equipment

1. Functioning IV line.
2. Patient-controlled analgesia pump.
3. For subcutaneous placement, an IV and infusion device attached to a subcutaneous butterfly needle or commercially available subcutaneous infusion port (Microsoft button).
4. Equipment for epidural placement would be provided by the anesthesiologist, who would ordinarily conduct the epidural placement.

Required Monitoring

All ICU patients receiving opiates, benzodiazepines, or phenothiazines should have frequent respiratory monitoring and hemodynamic assessments, including hourly measurements of blood pressure, heart rate, and peripheral oxygen saturation.

Required Laboratory Data

Baseline arterial blood gases.

PROCEDURE

1. Patient-controlled analgesia.
   a. Start an intravenous infusion.
   b. Instruct the patient on the technique.
   c. See Table 13-4 for usual doses and ranges.
2. Epidural opiates.
   a. Consult anesthesiology to establish the epidural placement.
   b. See Table 13-1 for standard doses.
3. Continuous subcutaneous infusion.
   a. Prepare the skin with betadine.
   b. Insert a 25-gauge butterfly IV line into the subcutaneous tissues.
   c. Secure the butterfly with a clear dressing. Alternatively, a continuous subcutaneous button may be inserted.
   d. See Table 13-1 for infusion instructions.

FOLLOW-UP

1. Review the hourly vital signs, particularly in patients on continuous infusions where agents might accumulate.
2. Document satisfactory analgesia. Record visual analog score every 8 hours.

3. Evaluate arterial blood gas results, peripheral oxygen saturation values, and the extent of respiratory assistance if any, required following drug administration.

DOCUMENTATION

1. Visual analog score every 8 hours.
2. Hemodynamic sequelae encountered as a result of drug administration.
3. Respiratory sequelae encountered as a result of drug administration.
4. Recommendations for adjustment of dosage based on the former three findings.

SUGGESTED READING

Gilman AG, Goodman LS: *The pharmacologic basis of therapeutics, hypnotics and sedatives,* ed 7, New York, 1985, Macmillan.

Hoyt JW: Pain management in the ICU, *Crit Care Clin* 6:295, 1990.

14

Interpleural Analgesia

Joan M. Christie, M.D.

INTRODUCTION

Interpleural regional analgesia was introduced in 1986 by Reiestad and Strömskag. The superiority of interpleural analgesia, compared with traditional epidural analgesia or intermittent nerve blocks, has not been established; however, the technique has gained acceptance in the management of postoperative pain following thoracic and upper abdominal surgery.

The mechanism of interpleural analgesia has not been well elucidated. Proposed mechanisms include

1. Diffusion of local anesthetic through the chest wall with block of intercostal nerves.

2. Diffusion of drug to the paravertebral area with block of nerve roots and sympathetic ganglia.

3. Direct action on pleural nerve endings. Contrast material injected through the interpleural catheter has been shown to spread throughout the entire pleural space, a fact that supports this proposed mechanism of action.

OBJECTIVE

To provide analgesia through an indwelling inter-pleural catheter following thoracic or upper abdominal surgery.

Indications

1. Postoperative pain following thoracic or upper abdominal surgery, such as renal or pancreatic procedures, cholecystectomy, thoracotomy, splenectomy, and hepatic resection.
2. Pain secondary to traumatic injury of the chest, including multiple rib fractures, sternal fractures, and soft tissue disruption of the chest wall.
3. Pain of oncologic origin, such as nonresectable lung or pancreatic cancer with intractable pain.

Contraindications

Absolute contraindications are

1. Infection at the site of injection.
2. Anticoagulation with elevated prothrombin time (PT) or partial thromboplastin time (PTT).

The following are relative contraindications.

1. Empyema can be a factor. Local anesthetic is less effective in abscess cavities secondary to pH effects. More rapid systemic absorption of local anesthetic from the pleural space has been shown in patients with empyema.
2. The presence of an indwelling thoracostomy tube that could not be intermittently clamped. The thoracostomy tube would be expected to drain most of the instilled local anesthetic, thereby reducing its effectiveness. If the thoracostomy tube can be intermittently

clamped, interpleural analgesia may still be an appropriate choice and can even be administered through the chest tube.

3. Bilateral chest disease requiring two catheters. Dual catheters have been used to provide analgesia for both sides of the chest. Large amounts of local anesthetic are necessary, and systemic local anesthetic toxicity is a potential problem. An epidural technique is probably preferable for bilateral disease.

4. Inability to place the catheter secondary to fibrosis of the pleura, a situation that may hinder successful insertion of small catheters.

PREPARATION

Equipment

1. A 17-gauge Tuohy epidural needle.
2. Sterile prep, drape, and gloves.
3. Ten milliliters of 1% lidocaine in a 10-mL syringe.
4. A 10-mL glass syringe.
5. Epidural catheter.
6. Preservative-free bupivacaine, 25 mL, 0.25%.
7. Size 4–0 nylon suture.
8. Clear occlusive wound dressing.

Required Monitoring

1. Electrocardiogram.
2. Blood pressure cuff.
3. Pulse oximeter.

Required Laboratory Data

1. Coagulation profile including PT, PTT, and platelet count.
2. Chest roentgenogram.

PROCEDURE

1. Obtain informed consent from the patient.

2. Obtain a visual analogue pain score (VAS) by asking the patient to assign a number to his/her pain, ranging from 0 to 10, with 0 being no pain, and 10 being the worst pain.

3. Place the patient in a sitting position with the arms folded and resting on a table (Fig 14–1).

4. Locate the fifth intracostal space posteriorly. Palpate the angle of the scapulae, which is found at the level of the seventh rib, and move up two rib spaces in the midaxillary line. Mark the fifth interspace (see Fig 14–1).

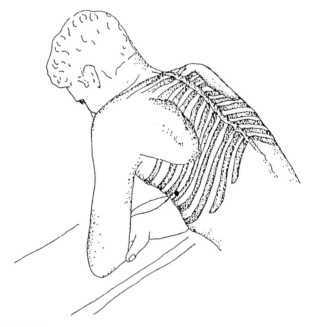

FIG 14–1.
Positioning for catheter placement. The patient should be made comfortable for the procedure. The sitting position facilitates insertion and is well accepted by patients. Note the mark *(black dot)* in the fifth interspace, denoting the insertion site for the Tuohy needle.

5. Wear gloves and prepare the skin over the fifth interspace with betadine; apply a sterile drape.

6. Place a skin wheal of local anesthetic, and continue the infiltration into the muscles just below the skin.

7. Advance the Tuohy needle through the skin in a plane that permits it to make contact with the superior border of the fifth thoracic rib. Take care not to advance the needle near the inferior border of any rib, as the neurovascular bundle is exposed at this level, and trauma could occur.

8. Attach a glass syringe containing 10 mL of air to the Tuohy needle, and walk the needle off the superior border of the rib. The negative pressure in the pleural space will draw the syringe plunger inward, or a loss of resistance will be appreciated as the plunger is advanced.

9. When the Tuohy needle is in position with good loss of resistance, perform an aspiration to ensure that the tip of the needle is not in a blood vessel.

10. Give a 10-mL test dose of bupivacaine, 0.25%, through the Tuohy needle, and observe the patient for 5 minutes for signs of systemic local anesthetic toxicity. Such signs might include dizziness, ringing in the ears, or metallic taste in the mouth.

11. Thread an epidural catheter 6 to 7 cm inside the space.

12. Withdraw the needle.

13. Secure the catheter in place with a size 4–0 nylon suture.

14. Aspirate the catheter and instill an additional 15 mL of 0.25% preservative-free bupivacaine.

15. Again observe the patient for signs of systemic local anesthetic toxicity.

16. Apply a clear occlusive dressing, and secure the external end of the interpleural catheter to the skin with tape.

17. If a continuous infusion is planned, connect the catheter to the infusion device tubing.

18. If an intermittent injection technique is planned,

place a filter capable of extracting particulate matter on the connector, and cap the system with a sterile blank port.

19. Label the catheter "Interpleural Catheter."

20. After catheter placement a chest roentgenogram should be taken to confirm correct placement. If the epidural catheter used is not radiopaque, inject the catheter system with 0.5 mL of contrast material to permit an adequate radiographic study of placement.

21. Dosing of interpleural catheters depends on the location of the pain. Dosage varies among patients. Dependent lung areas will have the most dense block, and higher areas in the chest wall may require a larger volume of local anesthetic to achieve analgesia. Positioning the patient with the affected side down permits gravity to help spread the anesthetic to the desired location. Monitoring of serum levels may be helpful to keep doses subtoxic. Seizure activity has been reported with blood levels of bupivacaine greater than 4 µg/mL and as low as 2.3 to 3 µg/mL.

Intermittent. Twenty to 25 mL of 1% lidocaine or 0.25% bupivacaine can be safely given as an intermittent bolus every 4 hours. If analgesia is incomplete and higher boluses are required, serum levels should be monitored.

Continuous infusions. Infusions of up to 1.25 mL/ kg/hr of 0.25% bupivacaine have been well tolerated. A loading dose of 0.5 mL/kg should be administered prior to beginning the infusion.

FOLLOW-UP

1. Check the pleural catheter daily. Ensure that connections are tight and that the catheter is not kinked or obstructed.

2. Assess the degree of analgesia by means of a VAS.

3. Evaluate the wound for signs of infection daily.

4. Obtain a chest roentgenogram every 3 days.

5. At the time of its removal, inspect the catheter to ensure that it is intact.

COMPLICATIONS

1. Incorrect placement of the catheter should be evident in the postplacement chest roentgenogram. In addition, appropriate analgesic effect would be lacking.

2. Pneumothorax.

3. Intravascular injection of local anesthetic with systemic toxicity.

4. Systemic toxicity from pleural absorption of local anesthetic. Toxicity is more likely to occur in patients who have concomitant chest infections, with more rapid absorption of the local anesthetic.

5. Horner's syndrome. Sympathetic blockade may occur secondary to local absorption by the sympathetic ganglion chain that lies adjacent to the thoracic vertebral bodies just beneath the parietal pleura.

DOCUMENTATION

The patient record should reflect the following information:

1. The cause of the pain being treated.

2. The VAS pain scale score from 0 to 10, before and after catheter placement and dosing.

3. The technique employed.

4. The size of the epidural catheter and Tuohy needle used.

5. The number of attempts at tube placement.

6. Any complications encountered.

7. Findings of the postcatheter placement chest roentgenogram.

8. An outline of the analgesic plan, to include suggested dosing intervals.

9. An order for vital signs every 4 hours.

10. Documentation of opiate and other analgesic use daily after catheter placement.

SUGGESTED READING

Fineman SP: Long-term post-thoracotomy cancer pain management with interpleural bupivacaine, *Anesth Analg* 68:694, 1989.

Laurito CE et al: Continuous infusion of interpleural bupivacaine maintains effective analgesia after cholecystectomy, *Anesth Analg* 72:516, 1991.

Raj P: Intrapleural anesthesia-applications and contraindications, *Anesthesiol Alert* 1:1, 1988.

Reiestad F, Strömskag KE: Interpleural catheter in the management of postoperative pain: preliminary report, *Reg Anesth* 11:89, 1986.

Stevens DS, Edwards WT: Management of pain in the critically ill, *J Intensive Care Med* 5:258, 1990.

15

Nasoenteric Feeding Tube Placement

Roy D. Cane, M.B.B.Ch., F.F.A.(S.A.)

INTRODUCTION

Placement of feeding tubes by the nasal route is a necessary and usually innocuous procedure. However, the increased use of small-caliber tubes for nasoenteral placement has been associated with a significant increase in intrapulmonary placement. The most common complication from intrapulmonary placement of nasoenteric tubes is pneumothorax. If incorrect placement is not detected, and intrapulmonary feeding is undertaken, lung abscess formation, empyema, acute lung injury, and death can ensue.

OBJECTIVE

To place and secure a nasoenteric tube.

Indications

1. Provision of nutritional support by the enteral route.
2. Provision of route for administration of oral medications in patients who are unable to cooperate and swallow on command.

Contraindications

Blind nasal passage of a nasoenteric tube should not be performed in patients with suspected or documented

1. Fractures of the nasal bones.
2. Suspected fracture of the base of the skull.
3. Esophageal rupture or stricture.
4. Coagulopathy.
5. Ingestion of caustic solutions.

PREPARATION

Equipment

1. Nasoenteral tube.
2. Lubricant.
3. Topical vasoconstrictor solution, such as 0.25% phenylephrine.
4. Topical anesthetic solution, for example, 1% to 2% Lidocaine.
5. Tape.

Required Monitoring

1. Electrocardiogram.
2. Pulse oximeter.

Required Laboratory Data

Coagulation profile including prothrombin time, partial thromboplastin time, and platelet count.

PROCEDURE

1. Introduce yourself and explain to the patient why the procedure is necessary and what you are about to do.

2. If the patient is conscious or reacts to noxious stimuli, anesthetize the nasal passage by gently introducing a cotton-tipped swab soaked in lidocaine solution. Wait 2 to 3 minutes for topical anesthesia to be achieved.

3. Similarly, vasoconstrict the nasal mucosal vessels by placing a swab soaked in phenylephrine through the nares.

4. Hold the tip of the nasoenteric tube at the patient's earlobe and mark on the tube the distance from the earlobe to the xiphoid cartilage (Fig 15–1).

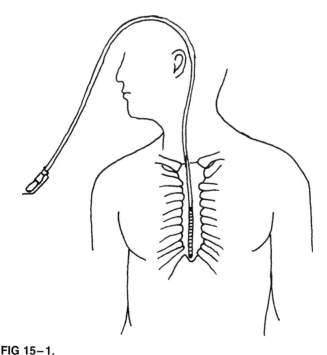

FIG 15–1.
To determine the depth for initial passage of the feeding tube, lay the feeding tube on the patient's chest with the tip of the tube at the xiphoid. Mark the distance from the tip of the tube to the ear.

5. Lubricate the nasogastric/nasoenteric tube and gently introduce it through the nares. Pass the tube along the floor of the nose. If the patient is cooperative, ask him/her to swallow as the tube passes through the choanae. Continue to advance the tube until you reach the mark on the nasoenteric tube. If resistance is met, or the patient coughs or complains of dyspnea, remove the tube and try again.

6. Obtain a chest roentgenogram and inspect for deviation of the tube to the right or left; deviation is indicative of probable endobronchial placement. With proper esophageal placement, the tube will be centered and pointing straight down (Fig 15–2).

7. If the tube deviates to right or left, remove it and try again (Figs 15–3 and 15–4). If the tube lies in the midline with the tip below the level of the carina, you

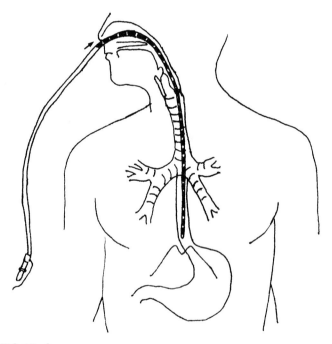

FIG 15–2.
Correct position of the feeding tube after passage to the depth measured in step 4. Note that the tube lies in the midline with the tip at the lower end of the esophagus.

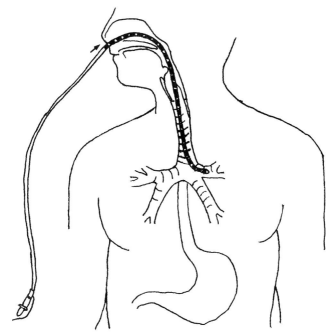

FIG 15–3.
Incorrect position of the feeding tube after passage to the depth measured in step 4. Note that the tip of the tube deviates to the right of the midline secondary to improper positioning in the trachea and right mainstem bronchus.

can safely advance the tube into the stomach or duodenum and secure the tube by taping it to the nose or skin over the maxilla.

8. Obtain another roentgenogram to confirm gastric/duodenal tube placement (Fig 15–5).

9. **Do not begin feeding or introduction of medications into the tube before checking the final tube placement with a roentgenogram.**

FOLLOW-UP

1. If a daily chest roentgenogram has been obtained, confirm tube placement.

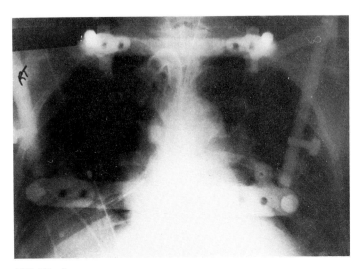

FIG 15–4.
Chest roentgenogram showing the tip of a feeding tube lying in the right bronchus.

2. Examine nose and face for signs of sinusitis or evidence of pressure necrosis of the nares.

COMPLICATIONS

The overall risk of the following complications from nasoenteric feeding tube placement is low. Complications can include

1. Epistaxis.
2. Cardiac arrhythmias.
3. Sinusitis.
4. Endobronchial tube placement.

Factors that predispose to tube misplacement and consequent pulmonary complications, include the following.
    a. *Endotracheal intubation or tracheostomy.* These procedures are associated with the most common risk and occur in 60% of those patients who

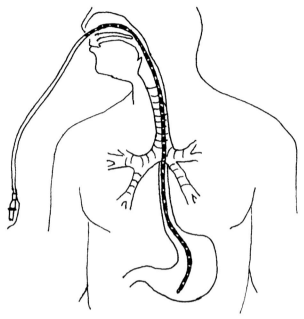

FIG 15—5.
Correct position of the feeding tube with the tube passing down the midline and the tip of the tube lying in the stomach.

develop complications of nasoenteric tube placement. Endotracheal or tracheostomy tubes can prevent glottic closure, impair the swallowing mechanism, and lead to endobronchial placement.

b. *Impaired neurological status.* This condition may result in diminished airway protective reflexes (gag, swallow, cough), which can lead to intrapulmonary feeding tube placement without the patient showing any signs of distress (cough, dyspnea, chest discomfort).

c. *Size and length of tube placed into the pulmonary tree.* Placement of larger caliber tubes (such as a nasogastric tube) in a main stem or lobar bronchus does not usually cause bronchial rupture, because the larger divisions of the airway are well supported by cartilage and smooth muscle. However, small-caliber nasoenteric tubes can be advanced farther into the bronchial tree before the tube size exceeds the size of the bronchus, thus the possibility of bronchial rupture and pneumothorax is increased. Chest tube placement is often necessary when these events occur. Clinical experience has shown that all small-caliber tubes, with or without stylets, are equally likely to be misplaced.

Common misconceptions about feeding tube placement include the following.

(1) *The cuff of the endotracheal or tracheostomy tube protects against intrapulmonary feeding tube placement.* Low-pressure cuffs on endotracheal and tracheostomy tubes allow easy passage of the small, pliable, lubricated feeding tubes into the lung.

(2) *Auscultation of a rush of air over the stomach area while air is being injected into the nasoenteric tube guarantees proper tube placement.* Transmission of sound generated in the lung to the stomach, and vice versa, is common and can be very misleading.

(3) *The tip of the nasoenteric tube overlying the gastric air bubble on a roentgenogram is confirmation of correct tube placement.* Roentgenograms are two-dimensional and cannot allow discrimination between a feeding tube lying posteriorly in the left lower lobe of the lung or in the stomach. Close attention must be given to the course of the feeding tube as it passes through the chest.

DOCUMENTATION

Documentation should include

1. Indication for tube placement.
2. Technique employed, with description of roentgenographic findings during and after tube placement.
3. Size and make of tube placed.
4. Number of attempts at tube placement.
5. Any complications encountered during tube placement.
6. Signature of person who performed the procedure.

SUGGESTED READING

Hendry PJ et al: Bronchopleural complications of nasogastric feeding tubes, *Crit Care Med* 14:892–894, 1986

Roubenoff R et al: Pneumothorax due to nasogastric feeding tubes: report of four cases, review of the literature, and recommendations for prevention, *Arch Intern Med* 149:184–188, 1989.

Roubenoff R et al: The technique of avoiding feeding tube misplacement, *J Crit Illness* 4:75–79, 1989.

16

Intravenous Hyperalimentation

Robert M. Craig, M.D.
Daniel R. Ganger, M.D.

INTRODUCTION

The goal of nutritional support is the restoration and maintenance of an adequate nutritional status. Nutrient deficiencies can lead to malnutrition, which necessitates nutritional support. Nutrient deficiencies (Table 16–1) may develop as a consequence of

1. Impaired gastrointestinal (GI) tract function.
2. Catabolism of acute illness.
3. Loss of muscle function.
4. Psychological factors.

Intense nutritional support may be administered either enterally or parenterally. Enteral alimentation is preferred when GI tract function is adequate (see Chapter 17, Enteral Feeding). Intravenous hyperalimentation (IVH) is the provision of the total nutritional needs

TABLE 16–1.
Pathophysiology of Nutrient Deficits

Inadequate gastrointestinal tract
  Acute abdominal trauma
  Problems with deglutition
  Motility problems of stomach, small bowel, colon
  Esophageal stricture
  Superior mesenteric artery syndrome
  Radiation enteritis
  Intestinal obstruction
  Short bowel syndrome
  Intestinal fistula
  Acute pancreatitis
Nutrient deficits related to metabolic consequences of acute illness and
  not to supply of nutrients
Obligate loss of muscle mass, not preventable by nutrient supply, such
  as neurogenic disuse atrophy
Psychiatric conditions
  Depression
  Anorexia nervosa
  Miscellaneous other problems

---

of the patient by the parenteral route. The major caloric source is concentrated glucose. Fat emulsion, amino acids, electrolytes, vitamins, and trace elements should be provided to meet the patient's total nutritional needs and to promote anabolism.

OBJECTIVE

Provision of a patient's nutritional needs by an intravenous route.

Indications

When the GI tract cannot be used, IVH should be considered for patients who manifest or are expected to

TABLE 16-2.
Possible Indications for Intravenous Hyperalimentation

Short gut syndrome
Irradiation enteritis
Small intestinal fistula
Scleroderma of small intestine
Intestinal obstruction
Postoperative adynamic ileus (if anticipated within 2 weeks)
Prolonged acute pancreatitis; pancreatic pseudocyst; pancreatic ascites
Inflammatory bowel disease: acute, chronic, fistulous disease; obstruction
Esophageal obstruction, until obstruction is relieved
Enteropathy associated with acquired immune deficiency syndrome
Thermal injury
Premature infants

manifest nutritional depletion. Examples of indications for use of IVH are listed in Table 16-2.

Contraindications

Intravenous hyperalimentation is contraindicated in

1. Uncooperative patients in whom a central venous line cannot be safely introduced or maintained.
2. Medically hopeless circumstances in which patient survival is not expected.
3. Patients in whom placement of a central venous line is contraindicated (see Chapter 2).

Relative contraindications to IVH are

1. Patients with metastatic or far advanced cancer.
2. Situations in which the GI tract is functional.

Despite the presence of a functional GI tract, IVH may be continued for patient convenience rather than instituting enteral nutrition. Furthermore, there may be occasions when the total nutritional needs of the patient can best be provided by a combination of both the enteral and parenteral routes.

PREPARATION

A nutritional assessment is required before initiating therapy to determine

1. If nutritional support is indicated.
2. Whether enteral or parenteral alimentation is more appropriate.

Timing of initiation of IVH is important, as most patients with temporary loss of GI function do not require IVH. A reasonable rule-of-thumb for postoperative patients is to provide IVH when the GI tract is dysfunctional for 2 weeks (or is expected to be dysfunctional for 2 weeks). If the patient is nutritionally depleted prior to surgery, IVH probably should be instituted preoperatively. Controlled studies for postoperative patients support these recommendations; however, guidelines for other acute abnormalities of the GI tract are not as clear. Nevertheless, 2 weeks without feeding is a reasonable standard for most conditions. Considerable clinical judgement is necessary in other conditions to predict the value of IVH.

Equipment

No particular equipment is required other than that necessary for placement of a central venous catheter (see Chapter 2).

Required Monitoring

None.

Required Laboratory Data

The nutritional status of the patient must first be evaluated. Table 16–3 displays measurements commonly employed for nutritional assessment, of which the most important are those pertaining to protein

TABLE 16–3.

Nutritional Assessment

Measurement of body composition
    Fat—triceps skin fold
    Muscle-midarm muscle circumference
    Impedance plethysmography
    Whole-body potassium measurements
    Creatinine height index
    Body weight and recent weight loss
Visceral protein measurements
    Serum protein, albumin, transferrin
    Skin test reactivity to recall antigens
Measurement of specific nutrients
    Serum electrolytes: Na, K, Cl, Ca, P, Mg
    Micronutrients: Cr, Cu, Se, I, Mn, Zn
    Vitamins: prothrombin time, vitamin B_{12}, folic acid, vitamin D
Nitrogen balance

---

stores. Table 16–4 lists different methods of assessing total body protein stores, indicating the relative reliability of these tests and their ease of performance. Frequently, it is difficult to ascertain whether abnormalities of protein stores reflect diminished nutrient supply or are direct consequences of the underlying disease processes, as both may result in diminution of the test values.

Data regarding total body protein stores also provide important prognostic information; diminished total body protein stores correlate with in-hospital or postoperative morbidity and mortality. Hypoalbuminemia correlates better with poor survival than with nutritional status. These indicators of nutritional status also may be used to monitor nutritional restitution.

In practice, the anthropometric measurements of triceps skin fold and midarm muscle circumference are performed before therapy is initiated, but the other body composition data usually are not employed. Serum protein and albumin measurements are obtained before institution of IVH and during the course of treatment.

TABLE 16–4.
Methods for Assessing Total Body Protein Stores

Method	Reliability	Feasibility
Nitrogen balance	Fair	All hospital laboratories
Creatinine height index	Fair	All hospital laboratories
Total body potassium	Good	Only in research centers
Impedance plethysmography	Good	Many medical centers
Serum chemistries	Fair	All hospital laboratories
Anergy to skin test antigens	Fair	All hospitals

Several factors impair the reliability of routine techniques for assessment of nutritional status in the critically ill patient. The edematous condition frequently encountered in critically ill patients confounds anthropometric measurements. Serum protein dilution secondary to fluid resuscitation, and non-nutritionally-related loss of serum proteins, particularly in patients with sepsis, diminishes the value of measurements of serum protein concentrations in critically ill patients. Frequently the clinician has to rely more on common sense and careful evaluation of the patient's history and physical examination rather than laboratory measurements to determine the need for nutritional support.

The following serum and blood measurements should be obtained before initiation of IVH:

1. Potassium.
2. Sodium.
3. Chloride.
4. Carbon dioxide.
5. Glucose.
6. Calcium.
7. Phosphate.
8. Blood urea nitrogen.
9. Creatinine.

10. Alkaline phosphatase.
11. Aspartate transaminase.
12. Bilirubin.
13. Complete blood count, including platelet count.
14. Prothrombin time.

PROCEDURE

1. Place central venous line (see Chapter 2). To ensure delivery of adequate amounts of nutritional substrates and to minimize the risks of infection, IVH should be provided through a dedicated line, with as few interruptions as possible (for example, blood drawing, infusions of blood products, administration of drugs). However, exceptions are sometimes necessary when venous access is difficult and the patient's problems complex, such as following bone marrow transplantation.
2. Select the amount of calories, protein, fat, vitamins, trace elements, and electrolytes the patient will receive.
   a. *Calorie supply.* The amount of calories required can be estimated by the Harris-Benedict equation that relates age, height, weight, and metabolic activity to estimated energy expenditure. In general, optimal calorie supply for critically ill patients is approximately 35 kcal/kg ideal body weight/day (2,450 kcal/day for a 70-kg person). The usual calorie source is carbohydrate in form of dextrose. Table 16–5 lists calorie supply with different concentrations of dextrose. Although usually provided to prevent development of essential fatty acid deficiencies, fat is an alternative source of calories. Use of fat as a significant calorie source may be important in special circumstances.
   b. *Protein supply.* Critically ill patients require 1.5 to 2 g of protein per kilogram body weight per

TABLE 16–5.

Calorie Supply With Carbohydrate Source*

Dextrose Concentration	Calories/L	Calories/mL	Calories/Day at Various Infusions (mL/hr)					
			50	60	75	83	100	125
D40	680	0.7	840	1,000	1,260	1,400	1,680	2,100
D50	850	0.85	1,020	1,220	1,500	1,700	2,040	2,550
D60	1,020	1.0	1,200	1,440	1,800	2,000	2,400	3,000
D70	1,200	1.2	1,440	1,700	2,160	2,400	2,900	3,600

*If 500 mL of the glucose solution is used per liter of infusion, usually with 500 mL of an amino acid solution.

day, supplied in the form of amino acid solutions.

c. *Calorie-to-nitrogen ratio.* To ensure anabolic utilization of delivered protein, an appropriate calorie-to-nitrogen ratio is required. Patients with simple starvation need 200 kcal/1 g protein. The critically ill patient requires a calorie-to-nitrogen ratio of 120 to 150 kcal/1 g protein.

d. *Fat.* Provision of 8% of total calorie supply as fat will usually ensure sufficient delivery of essential fatty acids. Providing more than 60% of the daily energy requirement with fat may result in serum lipemia and a fat overload syndrome. A carbohydrate-to-lipid calorie ratio of 2:1 is reasonable for most patients. Five hundred milliliters of a 10% fat emulsion provides 550 kcal.

e. *Vitamins.* Different disease processes may result in specific vitamin deficiencies. Examples of commonly encountered vitamin deficiencies are listed in Table 16–6. If any specific vitamin deficiency is suspected, the appropriate vitamin should be provided to replete the patient. In general 10 mL/day of a multivitamin preparation will maintain adequate vitamin supply for the critically ill patient. Remember that vitamin K, commonly deficient in patients with hepatic dysfunction and biliary obstruction, is not part

TABLE 16–6.
Vitamin Deficiencies and Associated Clinical Conditions

Vitamin	Clinical Condition
Thiamin	Alcoholism
Riboflavin	Alcoholism
Pyridoxine	Alcoholism
Folate	Nonspecific critical illness
Ascorbic acid	Burns
Vitamin K	Biliary obstruction; jaundice; cirrhosis of the liver

TABLE 16–7.

Trace Elements to Be Provided With
Intravenous Hyperalimentation

Element	Daily Requirement
Zinc	4 mg
Manganese	0.5 mg
Copper	0.3 mg
Chromium	10 µg
Selenous acid	100–150 µg

of standard multivitamin preparations and must
be added to the IVH formulation.

  f. Trace elements. Table 16–7 lists recommended
amounts of essential trace elements that should
be provided with IVH.

  g. *Electrolytes.* See Table 16–8 for suggested
amounts of electrolytes to be added to IVII
solution.

3. Write a nutritional prescription that reflects the
desired amounts and composition of nutrients and a
solution delivery rate. Standard order forms are
employed to minimize errors when writing IVH
orders. Most hospitals use a standard IVH solution
for patients with no special medical problems.
Table 16–8 shows a typical standard IVH solution
order form.

4. Initiate delivery of IVH after confirmation of
appropriate placement of central venous catheter
by chest roentgenogram. Initially, a relatively slow
rate of infusion is recommended. Increase the
infusion rate slowly over a few days while closely
monitoring the patient for evidence of any
metabolic problems (see "Complications"). The rate
of infusion should not be increased until all
metabolic derangements that may arise are
corrected.

Special Medical Circumstances

Modification of the suggested nutrient requirements
is necessary for patients with specific medical prob-

TABLE 16–8.

Standard Intravenous Hyperalimentation Solution

Component	Amount
50% dextrose	500 mL
8.5% amino acid	500 mL
Potassium acetate	20 mEq/L
Potassium chloride	20 mEq/L
Sodium acetate	15 mEq/L
Sodium chloride	10 mEq/L
Magnesium sulfate	8 mEq/L
Calcium gluconate	5 mEq/L
Sodium phosphate	15 mmol/L
Heparin	1,000 units/L
MVI multivitamin	10 mL daily
Zinc	4 mg daily
Copper	0.3 mg daily
Cromium	10 μg daily
Manganese	0.5 mg daily
Selenium	100 μg daily
Vitamin K	10 mg AquaMEPHYTON (phytonadione) weekly

Administer solution at_____mL/hr

Fat emulsion_____%; administer by way of a Y connector into central line at_____mL/hr

lems. Table 16–9 is a list of special circumstances commonly encountered in critically ill patients.

The total fluid volume can be restricted by increasing the concentration of dextrose and amino acids and by infusing the solution more slowly. Fat can be provided by a 20% emulsion. Special amino acid solutions for acute renal failure (provides only essential amino acids) and portosystemic encephalopathy (enriched with branch-chain amino acids) are of equivocal value, as controlled studies have not confirmed their efficacy.

Abnormalities of serum electrolytes can be corrected easily with a change in the electrolyte concentrations in the IVH solution. Serial measurement of serum chemistries is used to guide therapy.

Overfeeding, especially with high-dextrose infusions, increases production of carbon dioxide (CO_2) and may

TABLE 16-9.
Modification of Intravenous Hyperalimentation Solutions Based on
Medical Problems

Medical Complication	Modifications
Congestive heart failure	Sodium and water restriction
Acute or chronic renal failure	Restriction of phosphate, magnesium, and potassium
	Fluid restriction
	Occasionally addition of more sodium chloride to facilitate dialysis
	Preferential use of essential amino acids
Hepatic failure	Fluid and sodium restriction
	Branch chain amino acid solution with encephalopathy
Respiratory failure	Less carbohydrate and less calories when weaning off ventilator
SIADH	Increased sodium chloride concentration with diuretics
	Demethyltetracycline

be disadvantageous for patients with compromised ventilatory function, especially when being weaned off a ventilator. Lipids are metabolized with a lower CO_2 production than carbohydrates, making an IVH prescription with a higher lipid component more suitable for patients with respiratory insufficiency. A carbohydrate-to-lipid ratio of 1:1 is advised for patients with ventilatory insufficiency. Overfeeding with carbohydrates leads to lipogenesis and laying down of fat. Lipogenesis produces 7 to 8 times the amount of CO_2 that would be generated by metabolism of dextrose for energy; the respiratory quotient, or amount of CO_2 produced per amount of oxygen consumed, is high.

Peripheral Venous Infusions of Amino Acids and Fat Emulsions

Central venous access is necessary for standard IVH because of the hypertonicity of the infusate, which invariably results in thrombosis of peripheral veins. Isotonic or slightly hypertonic infusions may be used peripherally, but they are limited in the amount of calories and amino acids that can be delivered. Peripheral venous infusions of amino acids and fat can be used to supplement oral or enteral feedings for short-term therapy. A reasonable isotonic prescription for peripheral venous infusion is 500 mL of a 3.5% amino acid solution plus 500 mL of 5% dextrose delivered at a rate of 125 mL/hr. Addition of a 10% fat emulsion, delivered into the same venous line via a Y-connector, at a rate of 42 mL/hr provides a total delivery of 1,000 kcal/day. Provision of other additives in the infusion greatly increases the incidence of venous thrombosis.

FOLLOW-UP

Intravenous hyperalimentation is monitored best by a nutritional support service, usually comprised of physicians, dieticians, pharmacists, and nurses. In the absence of a nutritional support service, IVH preferably is provided in an intensive care unit under the direction of an specialist aware of the indications and methods employed. The following should be done.

1. Evaluate patient daily with respect to the following.
   a. The type and volume of IVH solution given in the preceding 24 hours.
   b. The patient's clinical status.
   c. Laboratory findings.
   d. The development of any complications.
2. Obtain the following laboratory studies weekly.
   a. Potassium.
   b. Sodium.
   c. Chloride.
   d. Carbon dioxide.
   e. Glucose.
   f. Calcium.
   g. Phosphate.
   h. Blood urea nitrogen.
   i. Creatinine.
   j. Alkaline phosphatase.

    k. Aspartate transaminase.
    l. Bilirubin.
    m. Complete blood count, including platelet count.
    n. Prothrombin time.
3. Measure serum trace element concentrations biweekly or monthly.
4. Evaluate the patient's nutritional status by performing a nutritional assessment (see Table 16–3) weekly or biweekly. The most useful measure of nutritional status in the critically ill patient is nitrogen balance. The urinary urea nitrogen (UUN) represents most of the nitrogen lost per day. Determine the nitrogen balance as follows.
    a. Measure the UUN in a 24-hour sample of urine.
    b. Add 3 grams of nitrogen to the UUN to account for other nitrogen losses.
    c. Subtract the nitrogen lost from the amount of nitrogen infused.

A positive nitrogen balance of 0 to 4 g/day reflects anabolism at least equal to catabolism.

Most of the other body composition measurements are not useful clinically in the critically ill patient.

Much of the required follow-up monitoring is performed by the nursing staff. Most hospitals have a standard from for nursing orders for the general care of the patient receiving IVH. Table 16–10 shows an example of such a form.

Development of electrolyte abnormalities and metabolic complications of IVH require modifications of the IVH components to fulfill each individual patient's need. Careful record keeping, including quality assurance data, coincides with the daily management.

COMPLICATIONS

The complications of IVH can be divided into mechanical (related to the catheter insertion and maintenance) and medical. The major complications and their treatment and prevention are outlined in Table 16–11.

TABLE 16–10.
Standard Nursing Orders for Intravenous Hyperalimentation.

Check chemstix every 6 hours
If infusion rate has slowed, do not "catch-up" by increasing the rate of
  infusion
Obtain SMA 20, complete blood count with differential, serum transferrin
  level, serum magnesium level, and prothrombin time every Monday
Obtain SMA 6 every Thursday
Call physician for temperatures above 100°F
Change intravenous delivery tubing daily
Inspect central venous catheter site daily. Change transparent dressings
  as needed, at least once a week
Obtain measurement of serum copper, selenium, chromium, and zinc
  every 2 weeks

Mechanical Complications

The major morbidity from IVH is related to central
venous catheter insertion. (See Chapter 2 for more information on potential central venous catheter complications.) Surveys of IVH indicate that the misadventure
rate with central venous catheters correlates inversely
with the experience of the physician, suggesting that
the procedure should be performed by a few designated
individuals.

Clotting of the central venous catheter can be devas-
tating, as it may limit access sites, which are the life-
line for some patients with chronic bowel insufficiency.
Sometimes the clot can be lysed with fibrinolytic infusions, but often the line has to be sacrificed. The addition of heparin in the infusate lessens this complication. Patients prone to this complication may require
long-term full anticoagulant therapy with heparin or
warfarin.

Catheter sepsis is a major problem. Determination of
the source of fever in a critically ill patient is difficult.
Carefully evaluate fever prior to removal of a central
venous catheter. Investigate and treat possible urinary,
pulmonary, and gastrointestinal sources. Obtain peripheral blood and central venous catheter blood cultures. If no other reason for the fever can be identified,

TABLE 16–11.

Complications of Intravenous Hyperalimentation (IVH): Prevention and Therapy

Complication	Therapy or Prevention

Catheter insertion
  Pneumothorax
  Hemothorax
  Thoracic duct injury
  Brachial plexus injury
	Experience of inserting physician

Thrombosis of catheter	Add 1,000 units of heparin per liter IVH

Catheter sepsis	Careful aseptic technique with insertion.
	  Dedicated line for IVH; avoid other uses.
	  If no other source for fever, remove line.

Electrolyte disturbances	Watch for increased potassium and phosphate requirements early in course of IVH Careful monitoring of potassium, magnesium, and phosphate in patients with renal disease With low sodium, suspect SIADH
Hyperglycemia Hypoglycemia	Careful glucose monitoring, especially early in course of IVH Gradually increase rate of IVH administration Put regular insulin in IVH bottle Avoid long-acting insulin
Air embolism	Care in the institution of the infusion Breath holding when lines are opened Use of clamps when the lines are opened
Hepatic cholestasis Fatty liver	Avoid overfeeding Provide mixed carbohydrate: lipid calorie source Consider cyclic alimentation

remove the central venous catheter and send the tip to the laboratory for culture studies.

Medical Problems

The most common metabolic disturbance occurs with glucose. Hyperglycemia may occur in the absence of diabetes mellitus, and is easily treated acutely with subcutaneous regular insulin in conjunction with the addition of gradually increased amounts of regular insulin into the IVH infusion. Avoid use of long-acting insulins. Although some insulin may bind to the infusion lines or to heparin, the amount bound is approximately the same from infusate to infusate. Because glucose and insulin are given concurrently, the risks of hypoglycemia or hyperglycemia are minimized.

Many of the metabolic complications occur early in the course of IVH. Patients receiving IVH may have quite large requirements for phosphate that lessen with each day of infusion. Special attention to serum magnesium, phosphate, and potassium is necessary in renal insufficiency, as elevated levels can occur quickly if usual quantities are infused. Some situations, such as amphotericin B therapy, promote enormous renal losses of these electrolytes, and delivery of massive amounts of potassium and magnesium is sometimes necessary.

Slight elevations of the liver enzymes, alkaline phosphatase, and amino transferases are commonly seen during IVH; the pathophysiology of these changes remains obscure. Liver biopsies generally show only excessive fat and cholestasis, but sometimes fibrosis and cirrhosis occur, especially when the IVH is given for an extended period. It is difficult to separate the effects of the underlying diseases from those of IVH, as similar hepatic derangements are seen with inflammatory bowel disease or the short gut syndrome. Management of the problem is not clear; excessive calories, particularly derived from glucose, may be disadvantageous. The condition may be improved with cyclic alimentation, delivering IVH infusions only at night, then adding heparin to the central line during the day as is commonly done with home parenteral nutrition. These hepatic abnormalities are usually benign in the short term and are not a reason to terminate therapy.

DOCUMENTATION

Write a note in the patient's chart that reflects the following:

1. Indication for nutritional support, including the patient's nutritional status.
2. Rationale for choice of parenteral route.
3. Desired daily calorie and protein delivery.
4. Pre-infusion laboratory values.

Write the appropriate orders for the IVH prescription and the follow-up monitoring and care to be performed by the nursing staff. It is desirable to rewrite the IVH orders at least at weekly intervals.

Placement of central venous catheter should be documented as outlined in Chapter 2.

Write notes describing the patient's status; development of complications, if any; and progress with nutritional support at the appropriate intervals as suggested by the recommended follow-up procedure.

SUGGESTED READING

Feinstein EI: Total parenteral nutritional support of patients with acute renal failure, *Nutr Clin Pract* 3:9, 1988.

Hiyama DT, Fischer JE: Nutritional support in hepatic failure, *Nutr Clin Pract* 3:96, 1988.

McMahon M et al: Parenteral nutrition in patients with diabetes mellitus: theoretical and practical considerations, *J Parenter Enteral Nutr* 13:545, 1989.

Perdum PP, Kirby DF: Short-bowel syndrome: a review of the role of nutrition support, *J Parenter Enteral Nutr* 15:93, 1991.

Rombeau JL, Caldwell MD: *Parenteral nutrition*, Philadelphia, 1986, WB Saunders.

Sax HC, Bower RH: Hepatic complications of total parenteral nutrition, *J Parenter Enteral Nutr* 12:615, 1988.

Solomon SM, Kirby DF: The refeeding syndrome: a review, *J Parenter Enteral Nutr* 14:90, 1990.

17

Enteral Feeding

Daniel R. Ganger, M.D.
Robert M. Craig, M.D.

INTRODUCTION

The early use of enteral feeding in critically ill patients has been advocated. Unfortunately many patients have multiple problems that affect access to the gastrointestinal tract and absorption and digestion of nutrients. The intestine may lose significant weight after 24 hours if nutrients are not provided; this may have important clinical implications, because it is now known that the gut is an active metabolic organ. The integrity of the gut should be preserved to avoid increased permeability and the passage of enterobacteria into adjacent tissues and the systemic circulation. Bacterial translocation has been shown to occur in states of hypotension, prolonged fasting resulting in atrophy of the gut, and when total parenteral nutrition (TPN) is the sole source of nutrients. The early use of enteral feeding in critically ill patients should lead to reduced morbidity and less sepsis when compared to parenteral alimentation or starvation. Although some clinical trials support this argument, others have not been as clear. Nevertheless, enteral feeding is safer and more economical than TPN and probably should be initiated earlier in many critically ill patients supported with intravenous hyperalimentation (IVH).

OBJECTIVE

Establish early, effective, and safe enteral nutrition to provide all the calories, nitrogen (as amino acids, peptides, or proteins), and other nutrients (vitamins, minerals, trace elements) required by the critically ill patient.

Indications

1. Provision of required nutrients. The vast majority of critically ill patients will not be able to receive adequate oral intake. Hemodynamic instability, respiratory failure often with mechanical ventilation, and altered mental status can affect the patient's ability to be fed safely by mouth.

2. Preservation of gut integrity. Enteral feeding is indicated to preserve the gut mucosa from atrophy, maintain gastrointestinal function, and minimize risk of bacterial translocation.

Contraindications

1. Nonfunctional gastrointestinal tract.
   a. Avoid enteral feeding in the presence of intestinal obstruction.
   b. Adynamic ileus is a relative contraindication, as nutrient absorption may still be normal. Although the traditional instruction has been to avoid feeding when patients have no bowel sounds, absence of bowel sounds may only indicate a gastric emptying problem. The finding of abdominal distention, confirmed by dilated loops of bowel on an abdominal roentgenogram, is more reliable to identify those patients who will not benefit from enteral feeding.

2. Inability to access the stomach or small bowel. Usually a feeding tube can be placed by some method. Rarely, a jejunostomy cannot be placed during laparotomy, or nasoenteric tubes cannot be passed even with the help of endoscopy or fluoroscopy.

PREPARATION

Equipment

The equipment required relates to that necessary for enteral access. When the oral route is unavailable, enteral feeding requires the passage of a feeding tube into some portion of the gastrointestinal tract. The jejunum is the optimal site for enteral feeding. The stomach can be used. The following options are available:

a. Nasoenteric tube. (See Chapter 15 for description of placement technique.)
b. Nasogastric feeding tube. This can be passed in a manner similar to that employed for a nasoenteric tube. The frequency of disturbed gastric motility in the critically ill patient may limit gastric feeding.
c. Jejunostomy tube. Two options are available for placement of a jejunostomy tube.
   (1) Placement by the surgeon at the time of laparotomy.
   (2) Percutaneous endoscopic jejunostomy. Percutaneous jejunostomy tube placement is particularly suitable for patients requiring long-term enteral feeding.
d. Percutaneous endoscopic gastrostomy.

Required Monitoring

No monitoring is required for initiation of feeding. See Follow-Up for a discussion of monitoring during enteral feeding.

Required Laboratory Data

Obtain baseline measurements of serum glucose, electrolytes, blood urea nitrogen and creatinine, serum proteins, phosphorus, calcium, and magnesium before starting enteral feeding.

PROCEDURE

1. Determine the patient's energy requirement (see Chapter 16). The patient's energy requirements can be calculated by the Harris-Benedict formula and adjusted by a stress factor based on the severity of injury or illness. Energy requirement also can be measured by indirect calorimetry, considered by many physicians to be the most accurate method in the critically ill patient. The metabolic responses to acute stress and trauma—namely, increase in serum levels of glucocorticoids, cathecolamines, glucagon, growth hormone, and enhanced gluconeogenesis from amino acids derived from protein breakdown in conjunction with insulin resistance—favor glucose intolerance and hyperglycemia. Thus, the energy needs of the patient are less in the first 24 to 48 hours of an acute illness, and the total amount of calories provided to the patient should be approximately 80% to 85% of the estimated or measured energy requirement.

2. Select an enteral feeding formula. There are many commercially available enteral feeding formulas for the critically ill patient, including a good selection of specific products for particular clinical situations. The claimed advantages of certain products are probably overestimated and unfounded. The majority of products provide complete nutrition in terms of protein, carbohydrate, lipid, mineral, and vitamin composition. Different proportions of certain types

of nutrients discriminate products for specific clinical indications. Some institutions use a simple formula with modular additives customized for a particular clinical situation, for example, burns, but the vast majority use standard commercial formulas. Table 17–1 provides a partial list of different products categorized by the protein source and suggests some clinical indications for each product. The following description of the different groups of products provides a rationale for individual selection. The physician ordering a particular product should pay careful attention to its contents, as with any other medication prescribed.

a. *Proteins.* Most critically ill patients have a higher than normal protein requirement (1.2 to 2 g/kg/day). Provision of the total energy requirement with standard enteral feeding solutions will generally provide the protein requirement.

Protein absorption is a problem in a number of critically ill patients. Intact protein in the gut is degraded to peptides and free amino acids

TABLE 17–1.

Application of Enteral Feeding Products* Based on Nitrogen Source

Nitrogen Source	Clinical Application
Intact protein (Osmolite HN, Isocal HN, Traumacal)	First choice
Small peptide (Peptamen, Reabilan HN)	Diarrhea; hypoalbuminemia
Free amino acids (Criticare HN, Vivonex TEN)	Crohn's disease; needle jejunostomy
BCAA† (Hepatic Aid II)	Liver failure with encephalopathy
(Traum Aid HBC)	Trauma
Essential amino acids (Aminaid, Travasorb Renal)	Renal failure; no dialysis

*The list of available commercial products is only partial and does not indicate any particular preference of the authors or editor.
†BCAA = branched-chain amino acids.

before absorption. Small peptides (dipeptides and tripeptides) are absorbed more readily than free amino acids and may promote a decrease in gut permeability, as well as improve liver function and enhance clinical outcome. Current data are insufficient to enable identification of one of these products as superior to others within the same category. The majority of commercial products have 35 g to 70 g of protein per 1,000 mL. Available preparations provide the following forms of protein:

(1) Intact protein. This should probably be the first choice in most patients.

(2) Small peptides. Patients with hypoalbuminemia (< 2 g/dL) and diarrhea have been shown to have good tolerance for, and nitrogen utilization from, products that are rich in dipeptides and tripeptides.

(3) Free amino acids (also referred to as elemental feeds). Because of their thin consistency, free amino acid solutions may be administered through small-caliber jejunostomy tubes. In selected cases of Crohn's disease, elemental diets have been shown to be effective.

(4) Special amino acids.

  (a) Essential amino acids. These are useful in nondialyzed patients with oliguric or anuric renal failure. Patients on dialysis with no protein restriction can receive intact protein or a peptide-based formula.

  (b) Branched-chain enriched amino acids solution. This is useful in patients with liver failure and hepatic encephalopathy, although several trials have not shown dramatic results. Despite some improvement in nitrogen utilization, clinical outcome in multiple trauma patients has not been shown to be better

than that achieved with more
conventional products.

b. *Carbohydrates.* Traditional wisdom regarding
energy utilization held that patients mainly use
glucose as the primary source of fuel during
states of hypermetabolism (sepsis, trauma,
burns). However, administration of large
amounts of glucose have been shown to induce
hyperglycemia, hyperinsulinemia, decreased
lipid mobilization from fat stores, and increased
production of carbon dioxide (CO_2).

Most of the calories provided by enteral
feeding are in the form of carbohydrates.
Addition of fiber to enteral feeding to add bulk to
stools and decrease diarrhea has not been proved
beneficial in critically ill patients, although it is
believed to be useful for some patients with
glucose intolerance.

c. *Lipids.* Many of the enteral products provide 30%
to 35% of the calorie source as fat and contain
different types of oils in a mixture of long- and
medium-chain triglycerides to provide essential
fatty acid requirements. Some enteral feeding
products may be low in lipid, but the majority of
products have sufficient lipids to prevent
development of essential fatty acid deficiency.
Special circumstances regarding the lipid
component of enteral feeding include the
following.

(1) *Malabsorption.* Medium-chain triglycerides
(six to ten carbon atoms), which do not
require digestion and are absorbed
unchanged, are the preferred fat source in
enteral feeding when there is evidence or
history of malabsorption. Medium-chain
triglyceride oil cannot be used alone because
it will not meet essential fatty acids
requirements.

(2) *Burns.* Lower concentrations of fat (10% to
20%), restriction of linoleic acid, and

enrichment with omega-3 fatty acids (50% fish oil mixed with 50% safflower oil) have been suggested for the burn patient. It is believed that this formulation results in less diarrhea and faster healing.

d. *Osmolarity.* The traditional view that osmolarity is crucial and that hyperosmolar products are associated with more diarrhea has been challenged; the problem of diarrhea is multifactorial (discussed later). Dilution of formulas at the commencement of enteral feeding *no longer is* recommended. Rarely, a patient will be found to be truly sensitive to a hypertonic formula.

e. *Nucleotides.* The addition of arginine and other immune modulators to newer formulas (Impact) has yet to be proved cost effective in larger clinical trials. At present, it can only be said that these products have theoretical advantages.

f. *Vitamins and minerals.* Most products provide at least 100% of recommended daily allowances. Rarely vitamins need to be added, for example, in patients who are alcoholic. Electrolyte contents vary in the different preparations. Particular attention should be paid to sodium in patients with fluid retention problems. Potassium, phosphorus, and magnesium may need to be restricted in patients with renal failure.

g. Fluid requirements are generally met by products with a 1 kcal/mL concentration. If fluid restriction is necessary, products with higher calorie concentrations (1.5 to 2 kcal/mL) are available. Dilution of the enteral feeding solution to half or quarter strength when commencing feeding is discouraged; this practice unnecessarily delays provision of the required energy.

3. Select a mode of delivery for the enteral feeds.
   a. Provide the total amount of calories in a

continuous 24-hour infusion. Intermittent or bolus feeding is not recommended as the starting mode.

b. Set an hourly rate for the infusion pump. The initial rate for the continuous feeding mode is usually 25 to 50 mL/hr. Increase the infusion rate every 12 to 24 hours by 25 mL/hr until a rate that provides the total energy requirement is achieved. If the desired infusion rate is not tolerated, reduce the rate by 25 mL/hr until feedings are tolerated. After a period of several hours, attempt to increase infusion rate again.

FOLLOW-UP

1. Volume tolerance. Abdominal distention, increased residual gastric volume, and diarrhea indicate feeding intolerance. Gastric residual volumes should be checked every 4 to 6 hours, or more frequently based on individualized need. When residual volumes are higher than 50 to 75 mL, stop feeding for 1 to 2 hours and then reinstitute at a slower rate.

2. Monitoring of enteral feeding.
   a. Measure serum glucose, electrolytes, and blood urea nitrogen (BUN) 24 and 48 hours after initiation of enteral feeding.
   b. Measure serum glucose, electrolytes, BUN and creatinine, serum proteins, phosphorus, calcium, and magnesium at least once per week.
   c. The frequency of laboratory data monitoring can then be individualized. Once the patient is stable, the need for frequent monitoring decreases.

3. Achievement of nutritional goals.
   a. *Nitrogen balance.* One of the most important goals is the achievement of a positive nitrogen balance (> 0.5 g). Nitrogen balance is equal to the nitrogen delivered (amount of protein intake

in grams per 24 hours ÷ by 6.25) minus nitrogen excretion (urine urea nitrogen in grams per 24 hours + 4). A positive nitrogen balance usually implies that calorie and protein supply are sufficient. During the hypermetabolic phase of an acute illness, this goal rarely can be achieved; a nitrogen balance as close to zero as possible is acceptable.

b. *Anthropometric measurements.* Improvement in anthropometric measurements, such as weight or triceps skin fold thickness, rarely are useful in critically ill patients because third space fluid retention is common.

c. *Visceral protein concentrations.* Visceral protein concentrations, particularly serum albumin, usually respond too slowly to be useful as monitors of improvement in nutrition. Furthermore, they are subject to non-nutritionally related changes in the critically ill patient.

COMPLICATIONS

1. Misplaced feeding tube (see Chapter 15).
2. Clogging of the feeding tube can occur when medications are given through the feeding tube without flushing. Several techniques have been described to unclog tubes, including the use of mechanical devices (brushes) or the infusion of solutions containing common cola beverages and/or pancreatic enzymes. The most important factor to maintain the patency of feeding tubes appears to be compliance with recommended nursing procedures.
3. Metabolic complications.
   a. Hyperglycemia may develop in patients with previously known diabetes mellitus or secondary to the insulin resistance commonly seen in the critically ill patient, especially those with sepsis.
   b. The majority of commercial formulas rarely will

   cause dehydration, hyperosmolality, or
   electrolyte imbalances.
   c. Abnormal liver function tests, commonly seen
   with total parenteral nutrition, are unusual.
   d. High-carbohydrate feeding can precipitate
   ventilatory failure or delay weaning from
   mechanical ventilation secondary to increased
   CO_2 production. Overfeeding may result in
   lipogenesis, which further increases CO_2
   production. The mechanism is thought to be via
   an increase in glycogenesis. Production of CO_2 is
   less with the metabolism of fat than carbohydrate;
   therefore, in patients with ventilatory failure,
   particularly if there is pre-existing CO_2 retention,
   a higher proportion of fat (30% to 55%) as the
   second fuel source is preferred. Commercial
   products with lower carbohydrates-to-lipid ratios
   are available (Pulmocare, Traumacal). These
   products have not been shown to improve
   morbidity or mortality.
4. Aspiration pneumonia. Multiple factors appear to
   be involved.
   a. Previous use of antacids or histamine (H_2)
      blockers.
   b. Relaxation of lower esophageal sphincter.
   c. Poor gastric emptying.
   d. The supine position during feeding.
      Unrecognized large gastric residual volumes may
      result in vomiting with aspiration. Routine
      checking of residual volumes in patients fed by
      nasogastric or gastrostomy tube is recommended
      every 4 to 6 hours.
5. Diarrhea, seen in 10% to 50% of critically ill
   patients receiving enteral feeding, appears to be
   multifactorial in origin and associated with the use
   of antibiotics. It is important to rule out an
   infectious cause. When an infectious etiology has
   been ruled out, the therapeutic options available
   are as follows.
   a. Change the formula from intact protein to
      peptide.

TABLE 17–2.

Sample Enteral Feeding Tube Order Form

Date_____   IMPRINT

ENTERAL TUBE FEEDING ORDER FORM

A new order form must be completed for all formula changes.
Orders received after 7:00 PM will begin the following day.

1. Formula selection   (Check appropriate)

___Standard, high nitrogen   (Osmolite HN)   1.06 cal/mL
___Fiber, high nitrogen   (Jevity)   1.06 cal/mL
___High calories   (Magnacal)   2.0 cal/mL
___Semielemental   (Reabilan HN)   1.33 cal/mL
___Pulmonary   (Traumacal)   1.5 cal/mL
___Renal   (Replena)   2.0 cal/mL
___Hepatic   (Hepatic Aid II)   1.2 cal/mL

2. Dilution   (Check appropriate)

___Full strength
___Half strength
___Other

3. Administration   (Check appropriate)

_____Continuous infusion_____mL/hr
_____Advance by_____mL q 12 hours, to goal rate of_____
_____Intermittent_____mL, q_____hours

4. Fluid (additional water, optional)

_____mL q _____ hours.

5. Modulars (to increase specific nutrient density, optional)

_____Tbsp Propac, can   (protein supplement)   3 g/tbsp
       TF
_____mL Microlipid/can   (fat supplement)   9 cal/mL
       TF
_____mL Polycose/can   (carbohydrate supplement)   2 cal/mL
       TF
_____None

6. Monitoring:

-Verify tube placement. (upper abdomen and lower chest film)
-Elevate head of bed 30° to 45° during infusion and for ½ hour after
   feeding stops.
-Flush tube with 30 mL of water when infusion interrupted or finished.
-Aspirate for residuals q 4 hours nasogastric or gastrostomies only
   If > 75 mL, decrease infusion rate by half
   If residual continues to be > 75 mL, stop infusion, notify M.D.
-Weigh patient today and qd/qod
-Intake and output daily
-Use liquid preparations for medications via feeding tube whenever
   possible

7. Laboratory

SMA 7 B daily for the first 2 days.
SMA 20, magnesium next draw and q Monday
24-hour urine for urea nitrogen q Sunday.
Physician Signature_____

    b. Decrease the delivery rate.

    c. Reduce the fat content (10% to 15%) of the formula.

    d. An antidiarrheal agent such as paregoric (4 to 20 mL) or loperamide (2 to 4 mg) may be added to the formula to be infused over 6 to 8 hours.

    e. Dilute the formula to half strength to decrease the osmolarity. This commonly is done, but hypertonicity of the formula is rarely a cause of diarrhea by itself.

    f. Review the medications the patient is receiving, because laxatives may be administered inadvertently to patients: for example, sorbitol as a liquid vehicle, or magnesium in antacids.

6. Intolerance of feeding. Abdominal distention, nausea, and vomiting are a manifestation of poor tolerance to feeding and may require the interruption of enteral feeding. Use of prokinetic agents (metoclopramide, 10 mg to 20 mg up to four times daily) can be attempted but rarely is effective.

DOCUMENTATION

    1. Write orders for the enteral feeding prescription. Table 17–2 is an example of an enteral feeding tube order form.

    2. A note reflecting the nutritional assessment of the patient and the calculated or estimated energy and nitrogen requirements should be written in the progress notes.

    3. Document the position of the enteral feeding tube position by radiography before initiation of enteral feeding (see Chapter 15).

SUGGESTED READING

Alexander JW: Nutrition and infection: new perspectives for an old problem, *Arch Surg* 121:966, 1986.

Bynoe RP. et al: Nutrition support in trauma patients, *Nutr Clin Pract* 3:137, 1988.

Cerra FB. et al: Enteral nutrition does not prevent MOFS after sepsis, *Surgery* 104:727, 1988.

Fink MP: Why the G1 tract is pivotal in trauma, sepsis and MOF, *J Crit Illness* 6:253, 1991.

Hamaoui R. et al: Enteral nutrition in the early postoperative period: a new semi-elemental formula versus total parenteral nutrition, *J Parenter Enteral Nutr* 14:501, 1990.

Heimburger DC: Peptides in clinical perspective, *Nutr Clin Pract* 5:225, 1990.

Meredith JW. et al: Visceral protein levels in trauma patients are greater with peptide diet than with intact protein diet, *J Trauma* 30:825, 1990.

Moore FA. et al: TEN versus TPN following major abdominal trauma-reduced septic morbidity, *J Trauma* 29:916, 1989.

Skeie B. et al: Branch-chain aminoacids: their metabolism and clinical utility, *Crit Care Med* 18:549, 1990.

Wilmore DW. et al: The gut: a central organ after surgical stress, *Surgery* 104:917, 1988.

18

Intubation Including Fiberoptic Laryngoscopy

Michael T. Johnson, D.O.

INTRODUCTION

The first principle of resuscitation and life support is to ensure a patent airway. In intensive respiratory care, airway management is fundamental to support of pulmonary gas exchange. Endotracheal intubation is an essential skill for any physician responsible for critically ill patients.

OBJECTIVE

To establish a secure artificial airway.

Indications

1. Relief of airway obstruction.
2. Protection of the airway. Intrinsic airway protec-

tion against aspiration is potentially impaired in patients with central nervous system obtundation or laryngeal denervation.

3. Facilitation of bronchial hygiene. There are numerous disease states where spontaneous bronchial hygiene is inadequate. Blind nasotracheal suction of the nonintubated patient, while feasible, is not always effective and is potentially dangerous. Potential complications of blind nasotracheal suctioning include airway trauma, vocal cord edema, and precipitation of life-threatening arrhythmias. Placement of an airway reduces the risks and is frequently enables more effective support of bronchial hygiene than nasotracheal suctioning.

4. Support of ventilation. Although positive pressure ventilation can be delivered by a mask over the patient's mouth and nose for short periods of time, prolonged ventilatory support is provided most effectively by means of an artificial airway.

Contraindications

None.

PREPARATION

Knowledge of the upper airway anatomy is required for safe airway management. Before placement of an endotracheal tube, perform a thorough examination of the patient's head and neck—including assessment of the extent of temporomandibular joint mobility, state of the patient's dentition, distance from the hyoid bone to the chin, and the flexibility of the neck (do not assess neck flexibility in trauma patients unless the cervical spine has been cleared).

Once the decision to intubate a patient is made, the route and laryngoscopy technique to be used need to be considered.

Route of Intubation

An artificial airway can be secured by one of four different routes:

1. Trans-oral
2. Trans-nasal
3. By cricothyroidotomy (see chapter 19)
4. By tracheostomy (see Chapter 20).

This discussion will focus on endotracheal intubation by the trans-oral or trans-nasal route. Table 18–1 is a list of factors pertinent to the choice of the trans-oral versus the trans-nasal route. The choice of route for intubation is controversial. Most clinicians agree that emergency intubation should be performed by the trans-oral route. While anatomic and physiologic factors are pertinent to the choice of route in some patients, frequently the choice is based on physician preference.

1. *Specific indications for trans-oral route.*
   a. Emergent airways.
2. *Specific contraindications to trans-oral route.*
   a. Marked limitation of movement at the temporomandibular joints.
   b. Obstructing mass in the oropharynx.
   c. Mandibular fractures.
3. *Specific indications for trans-nasal route.*
   a. Temporomandibular ankylosis.
   b. Surgical procedures involving the oropharynx.
   c. Cervical spine arthritis.
   d. Fractured mandible.
   e. Trismus.
   f. Prolonged intubation. Nasotracheal intubation is preferred by many clinicians for cases of prolonged intubation if a tracheostomy is not performed. Opinions differ as to the upper limit of safety for the duration of oral or nasal

TABLE 18–1.

Comparison of Oral and Nasal Intubation*

Variables	Oral	Nasal
Ease of procedure	Apneic patient	Awake breathing patient
Nasal bleeding	No	Yes
Sinusitis	No	Yes
Patient comfort	Less	More
Need for bite block	Yes	No
Oral hygiene	Difficult	Easy
Accidental extubation	More likely	Less likely
Tube size	Larger, shorter	Smaller, longer
Suctioning	Easier	More difficult
Laryngeal damage	More	Less
Contraindications	Mandibular fractures	Coagulopathies
		Nasal cerebrospinal fluid leak
		Nasal sinusitis
		Nasal fracture

*From Gammage GW: Airway management. In Civetta JM et al editors, *Critical care,* Philadelphia, 1988, JB Lippincott, p. 200. Used by permission.

intubation. The nasotracheal tube is better suited for long-term intubation than the orotracheal tube for several reasons.

(1) Stabilization is easier.

(2) Patients frequently show greater tolerance of the tube.

4. *Specific contraindications to the trans-nasal route.*

  a. Coagulopathy or thrombocytopenia.

  b. Nasal leak of cerebrospinal fluid.

  c. Nasal sinusitis.

  d. Nasal fracture.

  e. Maxillary fracture.

Laryngoscopy Techniques

Laryngoscopy with a rigid instrument is employed in most instances. Fiberoptic laryngoscopy is useful for intubation of patients with limitation of neck flexion or mouth opening. Specific indications for fiberoptic laryngoscopy include the following.

1. History of difficult intubation.
2. Anticipated difficult intubation.
    a. Patient with a short, obese neck.
    b. Patient with buck teeth.
    c. Patient with micrognathia.
3. Upper airway trauma.
    a. Fractured mandible.
    b. Hematoma in the upper airway.
4. Abnormal airway anatomy.
5. Cervical or temporomandibular joint arthritis.

Laryngoscopy may be omitted in spontaneously breathing patients whose upper airway anatomy is normal, when an artificial airway can be placed by the blind nasal intubation technique.

Equipment for Intubation With Rigid Laryngoscopy

1. Laryngoscope handle with functioning batteries.
2. Laryngoscope blades with functioning light bulbs, both curved MacIntosh and straight Miller blades (Fig 18–1).
3. Endotracheal tubes of proper size.
4. Suction apparatus with yankauer and flexible catheters.
5. Syringe for inflating the endotracheal tube cuff.
6. Stylet.
7. Mask and manual resuscitator bag for ventilation.
8. Tongue depressor.
9. Oral airway.
10. Nasal airways.
11. Bite block.
12. Oxygen supply.
13. Magill forceps.

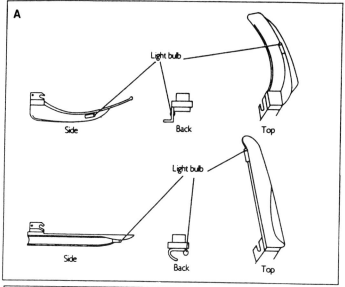

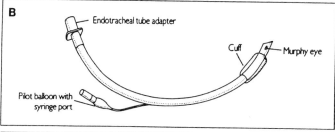

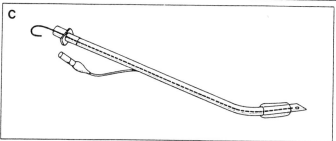

FIG 18−1.

A, the shape of the blade. The MacIntosh *(top)* is a broad, flat, curved blade with a tall flange for positioning the tongue. The Miller *(bottom)* is a narrow, straight blade with a curved channel in the center. **B,** looking for leaks. Before intubation, always check the inflatable cuff on the endotracheal tube and the pilot balloon and assembly, either of which may be the source of a leak. **C,** inserting the stylet. As you slide the stylet into the endotracheal tube, do not allow it to extend beyond the tip. After insertion, blend the tip of the tube slightly into the shape of a hockey stick. (Reproduced by permission of the artist.)

14. Adhesive tape or other means to secure the endotracheal tube.

15. Stethoscope to check proper tube placement.

16. Towels to position patient's head in the proper position.

Equipment for Intubation With Fiberoptic Laryngoscopy

Equipment for fiberoptic laryngoscopy is best kept on a dedicated, portable cart.

1. Ovassapian or Williams oral airway.
2. Olympus bite block.
3. Standard rigid laryngoscope blades with an assortment of endotracheal tubes.
4. Oxygen tubing.
5. Suction apparatus with flexible and rigid catheters.
6. Topical anesthetic spray.
7. Cotton-tip applicators.
8. Light source.
9. Lubricant.
10. Oral airway obturator.
11. Anesthesia mask with endoscopic port.
12. Antifog agent.
13. Three-way stopcock.

Required Monitoring

1. Electrocardiogram.
2. Arterial blood pressure.
3. Pulse oximeter.
4. Capnography, though not required, is desirable as it provides the most reliable means of verification that the endotracheal tube is in the trachea.

Required Laboratory Data

No particular information is necessary for intubation by the trans-oral route. Evaluation of the coagulation status of the patient is desirable before intubation by the trans-nasal route.

PROCEDURE

Orotracheal Intubation With Rigid Laryngoscopy

1. If the patient is conscious, explain why he/she needs intubation and what steps you will take to anesthetize the patient or airway.
2. Preoxygenate the patient with 100% oxygen for 5 minutes.
3. Check the endotracheal tube cuff for leaks and uniform distention.
4. Provide anesthesia/sedation. Anesthesia is necessary to blunt the reflex responses to manipulation of the airway (systolic hypertension, cardiac arrhythmias, bronchospasm, laryngospasm) and to ensure patient comfort. Lidocaine, 1.5 mg/kg, administered intravenously (IV) approximately 180 seconds before direct laryngoscopy minimizes airway reflex responses to intubation. Several options for anesthesia and sedation exist, including the following.
   a. Topical anesthesia of the upper airway.
      (1) If the patient has large amounts of oral secretions, consider administration of an antisialagogue, to reduce oropharyngeal secretions and to improve contact between the topical anesthetic agent and the mucosa. Glycopyrrolate, 0.1 to 0.2 mg IV, is recommended.
      (2) Sequentially spray the tongue, pharynx, larynx, and trachea with a solution of 4% lidocaine with a mechanical dispenser or a pneumatic aerosol. Alternatively, the airway may be anesthetized by having the patient inhale an aerosol of 4 mL of 4% lidocaine mixed with 1 mL of 1% phenylephrine (Fig 18–2).

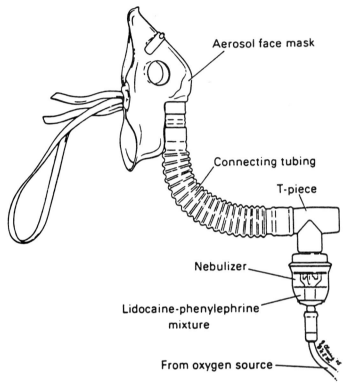

Aerosol face mask

Connecting tubing

T-piece

Nebulizer

Lidocaine-phenylephrine
mixture

From oxygen source

FIG 18–2.
Diagram of apparatus required for nebulization and delivery of lidocaine-
phenylephrine solution. Connecting tubing allows the nebulizer to remain
in the required vertical position regardless of the patient's position. (From
Bourke DL et al: Nebulized anesthesia for endotracheal anesthesia. *Anesthesiology* 63:690, 1985. Used by permission.)

    (3) When necessary, topical anesthesia can be
        supplemented with the following.
        (a) Superior laryngeal nerve block. Inject 2
            mL of 2% lidocaine beneath the right
            and left greater cornu of the hyoid bone
            (Fig 18–3).
        (b) Transtracheal anesthesia of tracheal
            mucosa and inferior aspect of larynx
            and vocal cords. Inject 4 mL of 4%
            lidocaine through the cricothyroid

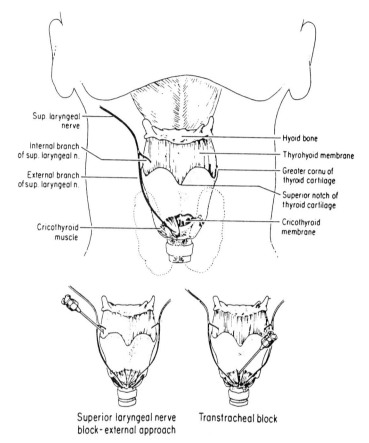

FIG 18–3.

Composite diagram of nerve blocks. Anatomy of the neck *(top);* needle placement for superior laryngeal nerve block-external approach *(lower left);* needle placement for transtracheal block *(lower right).* (From Reed AP, Han DG: Preparation of the patient for awake fiberoptic intubation. In Roberts JT, editor, Fiberoptics in anesthesiology, *Anesthesiol Clin North Am* 9:76, 1991.

membrane with a 25-gauge needle (see Fig 18–3).

Topical anesthesia is relatively contraindicated in patients at risk of aspiration.

b. Patient sedation (see Chapter 13). Depending on the patient's condition, a sedative, opioid, or combination may be titrated intravenously to achieve a calm, awake, spontaneously ventilating patient. Amnesia is a desirable adjunct to sedation. A combination of fentanyl (up to 1.5 μg/kg, IV) and midazolam (up to 0.03 mg/kg, IV) is recommended.

c. General anesthesia may be associated with apnea, aspiration of gastric contents, and hemodynamic changes. The risks of general anesthesia are usually greater than the risks of sedation and topical anesthesia.

   (1) Preoxygenate the patient with 100% oxygen.
   (2) Induce general anesthesia by IV titration with one of the following agents.
       (a) Thiopental (3 to 6 mg/kg).
       (b) Etomidate (0.1 to 0.3 mg/kg).
       (c) Midazolam (0.1 to 0.2 mg/kg).
       (d) Etomidate and midazolam may be associated with lesser effects on cardiovascular function than thiopental.
   (3) To facilitate laryngoscopy and intubation, paralysis can be induced with administration of a neuromuscular blocking agent after induction of general anesthesia. Neuromuscular blocking agents should not be given unless ventilation can be maintained with a face mask before intubation is accomplished. Succinylcholine, a depolarizing neuromuscular blocker, is recommended. A dose of succinylcholine 0.1 to 1.0 mg/kg IV, is usually sufficient in the critically ill patient. Succinylcholine is contraindicated if the patient is hyperkalemic or has suffered a recent denervation injury. Nondepolarizing neuromuscular blocking agents (vecuronium, atracurium, pancuronium) are alternatives to succinylcholine but should be used only by physicians familiar with these drugs.

5. Place the patient in the "sniffing" position by elevation of the head (approximately 10 cm) with a pillow or pad and extension of the atlanto-occipital joint. This position helps align the oral, pharyngeal, and laryngeal axes (Fig 18–4). Avoid exaggerated hyperextension (Fig 18–5).

6. With the laryngoscope in your left hand, insert the laryngoscope blade along the right side of the tongue, and move to the midline (Fig 18–6). To prevent the lip being caught between the teeth and laryngoscope blade pull the lower lip away from the teeth with your right thumb and index finger.

7. Advance the laryngoscope blade down the surface of the tongue with a slight lifting motion to expose the epiglottis (Fig 18–7). Glottic visualization is facilitated by elevation of the tongue and mandible along a plane approximately 45° above the horizontal. The primary glottic landmarks are the epiglottis and arytenoid cartilage (Fig 18–8).

8. Elevate the epiglottis to expose the vocal cords and laryngeal opening. With a curved laryngoscope blade, advance the tip of the blade into the vallecula; with a straight laryngoscope blade, lift the epiglottis with the tip of the blade (Fig 18–7).

9. Hold the endotracheal tube in your right hand and pass the tip of the tube between the vocal cords. Advance the tube into the trachea until the tube cuff disappears from sight to ensure that the cuff is below the larynx. The tip of the endotracheal tube should lie in the middle third of the trachea. The tube should not be advanced too far into the trachea, because it may come to lie in a bronchus, usually the right main stem bronchus.

10. If the first attempt at intubation is unsuccessful, withdraw the laryngoscope and provide oxygen and, if necessary, ventilation by a face mask and manual resuscitator bag. Evaluate why intubation was not successful. Improper position of the head

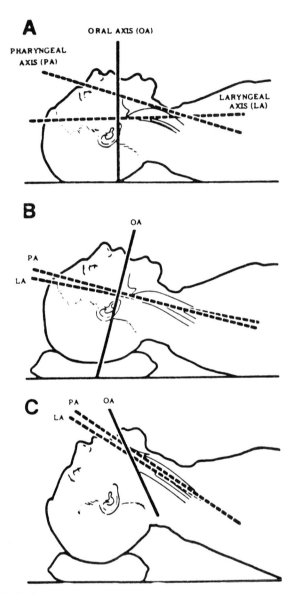

FIG 18–4.
Proper head position is important for successful orotracheal intubation. **A**, the oral *(OA)*, pharyngeal *(PA)*, and laryngeal *(LA)* axes must be aligned for direct laryngoscopy. **B**, elevate the head 10 cm above the shoulders with a folded towel to align the pharyngeal and laryngeal axes. **C**, extend the atlanto-occipital joint to achieve the straightest possible line from the incisors to the glottis. (From Gammage GW: Airway management. In Civetta JM et al, editors: *Critical care*, Philadelphia, 1988, JB Lippincott, p 200. Used by permission.)

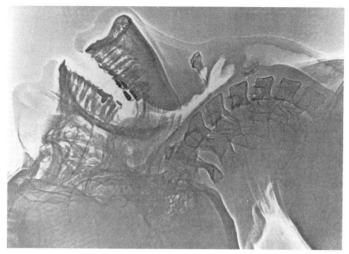

FIG 18–5.
Xeroradiograph of a healthy subject with head and neck extended. Note the marked angulation between the tracheal and pharyngeal air columns. (From Appelbaum EL, Bruce DL: Technique of tracheal intubation. In *Tracheal Intubation*, Philadelphia, 1976, WB Saunders, p 41.

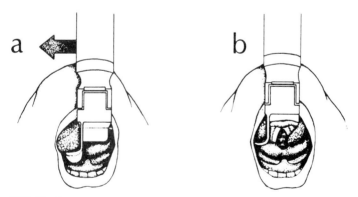

FIG 18–6.
Proper placement of laryngoscope blade: *a,* placement to the right initially, and then movement to the midline. This maneuver moves the tongue out of the way, *b,* depicts what happens if tongue is not moved to the left (hangs over and hinders passage of endotracheal tube). (From Shapiro BA et al: Establishing an artificial airway. In *Clinical application of respiratory care,* ed 4, St Louis, 1991, Mosby–Year Book, p 162. Used by permission.)

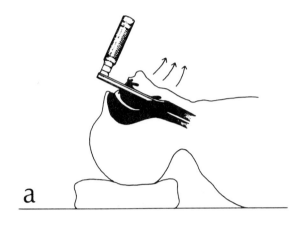

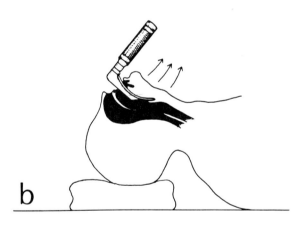

J GIANCARLO

FIG 18-7.
The laryngoscope in orotracheal intubation: *a,* shows the straight laryngoscope blade placed under the epiglottis to expose the glottis; *b,* shows the
curved laryngoscope blade placed between the base of the tongue and
the epiglottis. (From Shapiro BA et al: Establishing an artificial airway. In
Clinical application of respiratory care, ed 4, St Louis, 1991, Mosby–Year
Book, p 162. Used by permission.)

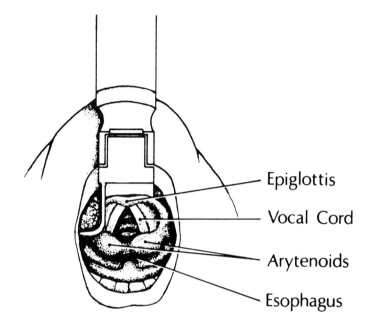

J GIANCARLO

FIG 18–8.
Primary glottic landmarks for tracheal intubation as visualized with proper placement of laryngoscope. (From Shapiro BA et al: Establishing an artificial airway. In *Clinical application of respiratory care,* ed 4, St Louis, 1991, Mosby–Year Book, p 162. Used by permission.)

and neck is the most common cause of failure of intubation. Correct the position of the patient's head and repeat steps 6 through 9. Attempts at intubation should not exceed 20 seconds.

11. Secure the endotracheal tube with adhesive tape. Be careful to avoid compression of the angle of the lips with the tube. A head halter is a dependable way to secure tubes (Fig 18–9).

12. Consider placement of a bite block in the mouth to prevent the patient occluding the tube by biting down.

13. Confirm proper tube placement. Auscultate the chest to ensure bilateral air entry. Tracheal tube

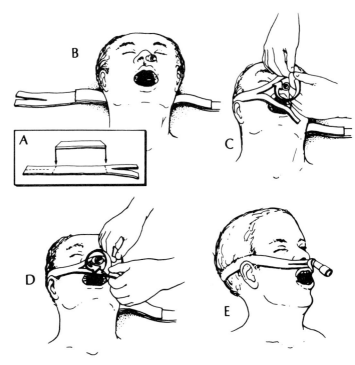

FIG 18–9.
The "head halter" technique for securing a nasotracheal tube. *A,* demonstrates how the tape is cut on both ends with the middle section apposed by a tape section so that hair will not stick to the halter. *B* shows the tape under the patient's head. *C* demonstrates how one side is brought over the ear and the top leaf is wrapped around the tube in a clockwise fashion. *D* demonstrates the bottom leaf wrapped around the tube in a counterclockwise fashion. The procedure is repeated for the other side of the tape. (From Shapiro BA et al: Establishing an artificial airway. In *Clinical application of respiratory care,* ed 4, St Louis, 1991, Mosby–Year Book, p 165. Used by permission.)

placement can be verified with capnography, if available, or by roentgenography of the chest and neck.

Nasotracheal Intubation

Placement of an endotracheal tube by the trans-nasal route can be accomplished with direct laryngoscopy, fiberoptic laryngoscopy, or without laryngoscopy (so-called blind nasal intubation). Nasotracheal intubation is more difficult and time consuming than orotracheal intubation and should be performed only by clinicians trained in the technique.

Nasotracheal Intubation With Rigid Laryngoscopy

1. The preliminary steps for nasotracheal intubation with rigid laryngoscopy are the same as outlined for orotracheal intubation (steps 1 through 5 in the preceding list). The nasopharynx and nares should be anesthetized with addition of a vasoconstrictor (phenylephrine, 0.25%) to the topical anesthetic solution to reduce epistaxis. Either naris can be used depending on nasal patency, but if equal patency is noted, the right naris is preferred because the bevel of the endotracheal tube will face the nasal septum during passage through the nose, thereby reducing risk of damage to the turbinates.

2. Once appropriate anesthesia/sedation has been achieved, place the patient's head in the sniffing position.

3. Lubricate a 7.0- to 7.5-mm internal diameter endotracheal tube with lidocaine ointment.

4. Introduce the endotracheal tube into the naris with the bevel of the tube flush with the nasal septum and advance the tube along the floor of the nose with consistent, gentle pressure. When the tube passes through the choanae, resistance to passage will diminish.

5. Once the tube is past the choanae, introduce the laryngoscope blade into the mouth and expose the larynx in the manner described above for orotracheal intubation.

6. Under direct vision, advance the tube and guide the tip between the vocal cords. If the tube tends to lie posterior to the larynx, gently grasp the tip of the tube with a Magill forceps and guide it into the larynx.

7. Once the tip of the tube has passed through the

larynx, advance the tube and position as described earlier. Check for bilateral air entry and obtain chest roentgenogram to confirm proper tube placement.

8. Secure the tube with adhesive tape (see Fig 18–9).

Blind Nasotracheal Intubation Without Laryngoscopy

Blind nasotracheal intubation is usually used when direct laryngoscopy, ventilation by mask, or induction of anesthesia before intubation would not be safe because the patient's airway could be lost.

1. Provide anesthesia. In most circumstances, topical anesthesia with addition of a vasoconstrictor to the nasal passages is the only anesthesia required.

2. Place the patient's head in the sniffing position.

3. Introduce the endotracheal tube through the naris in the manner outlined earlier.

4. Advance the tube into the oropharynx while noting air movement in and out of the tube. Breath sounds at the proximal end of the tube will be maximal when the tube is just above the glottis.

5. Once the tube is positioned above the glottis, rapidly advance the tube at the beginning of inspiration. The vocal cords will be widely abducted during inspiration, facilitating tube passage with minimal risk of vocal cord trauma. As the tube enters the trachea the patient will cough, unless the trachea has been anesthetized.

6. If movement of air through the tube ceases when the tube is advanced, it has entered one of the pyriform sinuses or the esophagus. Withdraw the tube until breath sounds are again noted and then repeat step 5.

7. If the trachea is not intubated with a second attempt, re-evaluate the position of the patient's head. Malposition of the head is the most common reason for failure of blind nasal intubation. Occasionally, the head may need to be repositioned with more or less cervical flexion, depending on the anatomy of the patient's neck and airway. Intubation may also be facilitated by rotation of the proximal end of the tube. Extrusion of the tongue moves the supralaryngeal structures anteriorly

and inhibits reflex swallowing. Extrusion of the tongue may facilitate blind nasotracheal intubation.

8. Once the trachea is intubated, secure the tube and check proper placement, as outlined earlier.

9. If intubation is not achieved after the maneuvers described in step 7, reconsider the choice of intubation technique. Fiberoptic laryngoscopy may offer a better technique.

Intubation With Fiberoptic Laryngoscopy

Fiberoptic laryngoscopy is more difficult and time-consuming than rigid laryngoscopy. The technique should be performed only by clinicians with appropriate training and experience.

1. Check the fiberoptic endoscope ("fiberscope") to ensure proper function. Check the adequacy of the light source.

2. Sedate the patient and anesthetize the airway as described for nasotracheal intubation with a rigid laryngoscope.

3. Position the patient. The sniffing position, used for rigid laryngoscopy, usually will place the epiglottis against the posterior pharyngeal wall and lead to greater difficulty in visualization of the glottis and passage of the fiberscope through the glottis (Fig 18–10). Therefore, for fiberoptic laryngoscopy, position the patient with no pillow under the head and the neck slightly extended. Extend the head at the atlanto-occipital joint. This maneuver will lift the epiglottis off the posterior pharyngeal wall (Fig 18–11).

4. Apply an antifog agent to the lens of the fiberscope. Adjust the focus of the lens before introduction of the fiberscope into the patient.

5. Lubricate the insertion tube of the fiberscope with a water-soluble jelly, beginning at the distal end and moving proximal to avoid the coating the lens.

6. Select the largest sized endotracheal tube that will

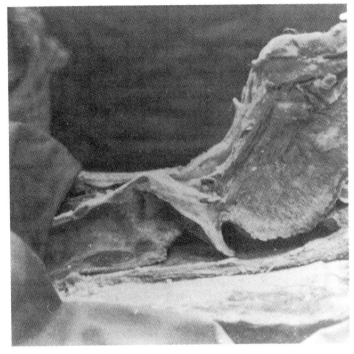

FIG 18–10.
Epiglottis in apposition to posterior pharyngeal wall during sniffing position. (From Roberts JT: Anatomy and patient positioning for fiberoptic laryngoscopy. In Roberts JT, editor: Fiberoptics in anesthesia, *Anesthesiology Clin North Am* 9:58, 1991. Used by permission.)

fit over the fiberoptic scope and pass easily through the patient's airway. Cut the endotracheal tube to the appropriate length because a shorter tube is easier to manipulate. Immerse the endotracheal tube in warm sterile water or saline to soften the tube. Pass the endotracheal tube over the fiberscope and position the tube at the proximal end of the fiberscope.

7. Run a constant flow of oxygen (3 L/min) through the suction port of the fiberscope. This oxygen flow helps keep the lens free of secretions, mucous, and blood and increases the patient's inspired oxygen concentration. A three-way stopcock, inserted on

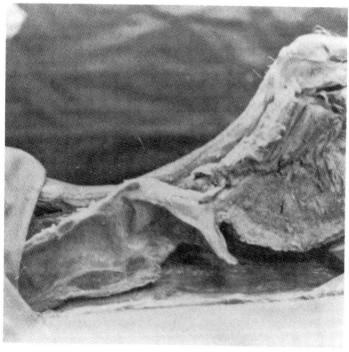

FIG 18–11.
Epiglottis separated from the posterior pharyngeal wall by cervical and atlanto-occipital extension. (From Roberts JT: Anatomy and patient positioning for fiberoptic laryngoscopy. In Roberts JT, editor: Fiberoptics in anesthesia, *Anesthesiology Clin North Am* 9:58, 1991. Used by permission.)

the suction port and connected to the oxygen source and the suction, allows the operator to switch between oxygen flow and suction as needed (Fig 18–12).

8. Grasp the controls of the fiberscope in one hand, with your thumb on the angle control and index finger over the three-way stopcock to control oxygen flow or apply suction. Fully extend the insertion tube of the fiberscope with the other hand and manipulate the angle control to ensure that the tip moves up and down and not sideways.

9. You are now ready to proceed with fiberoptic intubation by either the trans-oral or trans-nasal

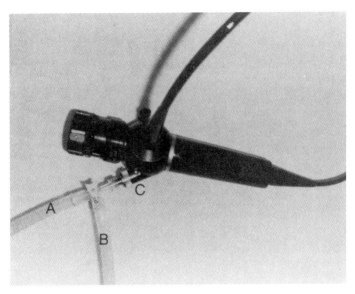

FIG 18–12.
A three-way stopcock allows alternate suction *(A)* and oxygen flow *(B)* through the suction port *(C)*. (From Patil VU: Oral and nasal fiberoptic intubation with a single lumen tube. In Roberts JT, editor, *Anesthesiol Clin North Am* 9:84, 1991. Used by permission.)

    route, depending on which route is best suited for the patient.
10. Trans-oral fiberoptic intubation.
    a. Insert either a Williams airway (Fig 18–13) or an Ovassapian airway (Fig 18–14) into the mouth in the midline. The Ovassapian airway has dorsal openings that allow the endotracheal tube be removed from the airway with minimal manipulation and without removal of the endotracheal tube adapter. With the Williams airway, the endotracheal tube adapter, must be removed prior to placing the endotracheal tube over the insertion tube of the fiberscope to enable removal of the airway after intubation is completed.
    b. Advance the fiberscope through the airway and

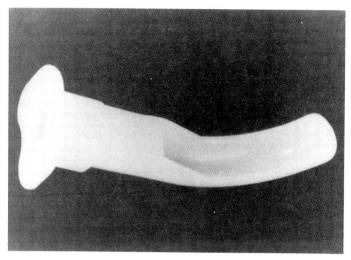

FIG 18–13.
The Williams airway guides the fiberscope and protects the fiberscope from injury by the teeth. (From Kraft M: Ancillary fiberoptic equipment. In Roberts JT, editor, Fiberoptics in Anesthesia, *Anesthesiol Clin North Am* 9:48, 1991. Used by permission.)

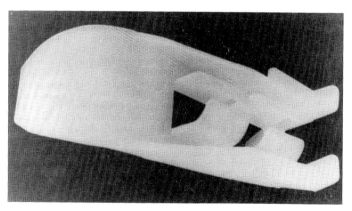

FIG 18–14.
The Ovassapian airway guides the fiberscope, prevents damage to the fiberscope by the teeth, and also may be easily dislodged from the mouth after intubation without removing the endotracheal tube adapter. (From Kraft M: Ancillary fiberoptic equipment. In Roberts JT, editor, Fiberoptics in anesthesia, *Anesthesiol Clin North Am* 9:49, 1991. Used by permision.)

into the oropharynx; take care to keep the fiberscope in the midline. Slowly advance and identify anatomic structures as you proceed. The depth of the adult mouth to the posterior pharyngeal wall is approximately 8 to 10 cm (Fig 18–15). Advance to this depth; you will be just past the end of the Ovassapian or Williams airway. Flex the tip of the fiberscope anteriorly; the larynx should be visible. If the larynx is not seen, advance the fiberscope further or slightly rotate the fiberscope to bring the larynx into view (Fig 18–16). If the larynx is still not apparent, the fiberscope tip is most likely not in the midline and the lens is facing the piriform fossa, oropharyngeal mucosa, or is in the esophagus. Withdraw the fiberscope insertion tube and check that the oral airway is in the midline position. Also, if necessary, clean the lens. Repeat this procedure until the larynx is identified.

c. Position the fiberscope tip so that the vocal cords lie in the center of field. Advance the fiberscope between the vocal cords into the

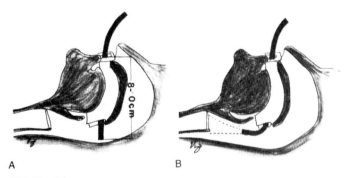

A   B

FIG 18–15.
Important steps in visualization of the larynx. **A,** position: midline, depth: 8 to 10 cm through the mouth. **B,** upward angle bend tip of fiberscope. (From Patil VU: Oral and nasal fiberoptic intubation with a single lumen tube. In Roberts JT, editor, *Anesthesiol Clin North Am* 9:86, 1991. Used by permission.)

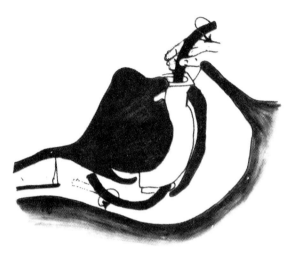

FIG 18–16.
Slight internal rotation of the insertion tube will guide the tip into the midline. (From Patil VU: Oral and nasal fiberoptic intubation with a single lumen tube. In Roberts JT, editor, *Anesthesiol Clin North Am* 9:86, 1991. Used by permission.)

larynx. Immediately after the vocal cords, you will see the thyroid cartilage; return the tip of the fiberscope to the neutral position and advance to view the tracheal cartilages.

d. Position the fiberscope tip above the carina. Advance the endotracheal tube over the insertion tube of the fiberscope into the trachea. If the endotracheal tube will not pass the arytenoids or aryepiglottic folds, rotate the endotracheal tube and displace the mandible anteriorly by further cervical extension.

e. Withdraw the fiberscope from the endotracheal tube. Verify proper placement of the endotracheal tube in the trachea as you remove the fiberscope.

f. Remove the Ovassapian or Williams oral airway.

11. Trans-nasal fiberoptic intubation.
   a. Insert the well-lubricated fiberscope through

the naris to approximately 12 to 14 cm. At this depth the fiberscope should not be in the esophagus and there should be enough room to allow manipulation of the fiberscope.

b. Direct the fiberscope in the manner described for trans-oral fiberoptic intubation and position the tip of the fiberscope above the carina.

c. Once the fiberscope is located above the carina, advance the endotracheal tube into the trachea as described previously.

d. Remove the fiberscope and verify endotracheal tube position in the trachea.

FOLLOW-UP

Following intubation, the immediate concern is to ensure that the tube is properly positioned in the trachea.

1. Inflate the cuff on the endotracheal tube and auscultate the chest and abdomen to establish that air entry into the lungs is equal and bilateral. Symmetrical ventilation should be ascertained by auscultating both lung fields for breath sounds at the anterior axillary line of the chest. Even if the patient is breathing spontaneously, give a few large positive pressure breaths with a manual ventilator while listening to breath sounds. Capnography can be used to verify tracheal intubation.

2. After the airway is secured, obtain a roentgenogram of the chest to verify tube placement in the middle third of the trachea (Fig 18–17).

3. Every 8-hour shift, check for the following.
   a. Bilateral air entry.
   b. Appropriate taping of the tube without undue pressure on the lips or alae nasi.
   c. Appropriate endotracheal cuff inflation. The cuff should maintain a seal with a lateral tracheal

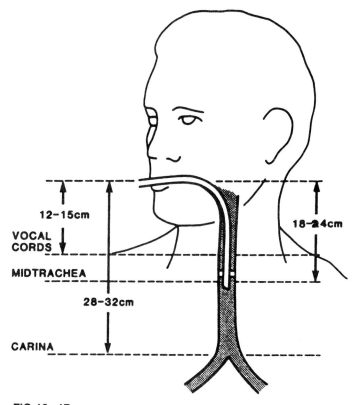

FIG 18–17.
Malposition of the endotracheal tube can be suspected from the depth of insertion. In an average adult, the 18- to 24-cm mark will show at the incisors when the tip of the tube is midway between the vocal cords and the carina. (From Gammage GW; Airway management. In Civetta JM et al, editors, In *Critical care,* Philadelphia, 1988, JB Lippincott, p 203. Used by permission.)

wall pressure of less than 25 cm H_2O to minimize risk of pressure-related complications. The goal of acceptable cuff pressure can be achieved either by cuff inflation with measurement of the intracuff pressure or by allowing a minimal leak to occur at peak inspiration.

4. Examine the patient daily for signs of sinusitis (purulent nasal discharge, erythema, edema and warmth of the skin overlying the sinuses).

COMPLICATIONS

Complications of tracheal intubation can be divided into three categories (Table 18–2), depending on when they occur:

1. During direct laryngoscopy and intubation.
2. While the artificial airway is in place.
3. After extubation.

TABLE 18–2.

Complications of Tracheal Intubation*

During direct laryngoscopy and intubation of the trachea
    Dental and oral soft tissue trauma
    Hypertension and tachycardia
    Cardiac dysrhythmias
    Inhalation (aspiration) of gastric contents
While tracheal tube is in place
    Tracheal tube obstruction
    Endobronchial intubation
    Esophageal intubation
    Accidental extubation
    Increased resistance to breathing
    Tracheal mucosa ischemia
Immediate and delayed complications after extubation of the trachea
    Laryngospasm
    Inhalation (aspiration) of gastric contents
    Pharyngitis (sore throat)
    Laryngitis
    Laryngeal or subglottic edema
    Laryngeal ulceration with or without granuloma formation
    Tracheitis
    Tracheal stenosis
    Vocal cord paralysis
    Arytenoid cartilage dislocation

*From Stoelting RK, Miller RD: *Basics of anesthesia*, ed 2, New York, 1989; Churchill Livingstone, p 170. Used by permission.

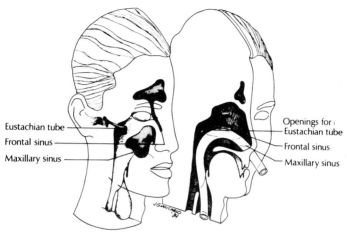

FIG 18–18.
Anatomic model showing where a nasotracheal tube may block frontal and maxillary sinus drainage and the eustachian tube. (From Shapiro BA et al: Establishing an artificial airway. In *Clinical application of respiratory care*, ed 4, St Louis, Mosby–Year Book, p 171. Used by permission.)

Nasotracheal intubation has unique complications, including pressure necrosis of the alae nasi, acute sinusitis secondary to occlusion of sinus drainage, and inner ear infection secondary to occlusion of the opening of the eustachian tube (Fig 18–18).

DOCUMENTATION

Write a procedure note in the patient's chart that includes:

1. Indication for intubation.
2. Reasons for choice of route and laryngoscopy technique.
3. Anesthesia/sedation employed, including doses of medication.
4. Size of endotracheal tube used.
5. Distance mark (in cm) on the tube at the skin surface.

6. Cuff inflation volume and pressure.
7. Findings of postintubation chest roentgenogram.
8. Complications, if any, encountered during intubation.

SUGGESTED READING

Applebaum EL, Bruce DL: *Tracheal intubation,* Philadelphia, 1976, WB Saunders.

Gammage GW: Airway management. In Civetta JM et al: *Critical care,* Philadelphia, 1988, JB Lippincott.

Roberts JT, editor: Fiberoptics in anesthesia, *Anesthesiol Clin North Am* 1991, pp 1–193.

Shapiro BA et al: Establishing an artificial airway. In *Clinical application of respiratory care,* ed 4, Chicago, 1989, Mosby–Year Book, p 153.

Shapiro BA et al: Maintaining and removing artificial airways. In *Clinical application of respiratory care,* ed 4, St Louis, 1991, Mosby–Year Book, p 177.

Shapiro BA et al: Laryngeal and tracheal complications of artificial airways. In *Clinical application of respiratory care,* ed 4, St Louis, 1991, Mosby–Year Book, p 195.

19

Cricothyroidostomy

Michael H. Albrink, M.D.

INTRODUCTION

Cricothyroidostomy is one of simplest and most basic airway maneuvers, yet it provokes considerable anxiety because it is often performed in emergency circumstances. Cricothyroidostomy is the most elementary of surgical airways and should be performed quickly, concisely, and efficiently.

OBJECTIVE

To place an artificial airway through the cricothyroid membrane in emergency circumstances where placement of an endotracheal tube by the oral or nasal route is either impossible or contraindicated.

Indications

Cricothyroidostomy is indicated whenever an emergency airway is necessary and conventional endotracheal intubation through the oral and nasal routes is either impossible or contraindicated. Examples of clinical situations where placement of an emergency airway may require cricothyroidostomy include

1. Edema of the upper airway (naso- and oropharynx) and larynx.
2. Suspected cervical spine injury.
3. Multiple trauma.

Cricothyroidostomy is associated with a lesser incidence of complications and can be performed more rapidly and easily than emergent tracheostomy in the acutely traumatized patient.

At some institutions, cricothyroidostomy is preferred to tracheostomy for prolonged airway management.

Contraindications

It is difficult to conceive of a situation where cricothyroidostomy is not indicated. If an artificial airway is needed in an adult patient, and other means of airway access are not applicable, a cricothyroidostomy should be performed. Cricothyroidostomy is considered to be contraindicated in patients under the age of 12 years, tracheostomy being the preferred method for these patients.

PREPARATION

Evaluate the patient to determine the following:

1. Does the patient need an emergency artificial airway? (See Chapter 18.)
2. Can an endotracheal tube be placed by the oral or nasal route?

If the patient requires an emergency artificial airway and cannot be intubated by more conventional means, proceed with cricothyroidostomy.

Equipment

1. Antiseptic solution.
2. Scalpel.

3. Single-curved hemostat.
4. Endotracheal tube or tracheostomy tube.

These tools are the only truly necessary equipment.

An endotracheal tube may be used in lieu of a commercially available tracheostomy appliance in urgent situations. If possible additional instruments such as hemostats, "cat's paw" retractors, and a Trousseau tracheal spreader may be helpful. In this often emergent and stressful situation, simplicity may be prudent. Commercially prepared cricothyroidostomy kits that usually contain an airway with a sharp trocar style introducer are available.

Required Monitoring

1. Electrocardiogram.
2. Pulse oximeter.
3. Arterial pressure monitoring is desirable. The hierarchy and triage of critical interventions (Airway, Breathing, and Circulation) seldom allow the luxury of this monitoring, because "airway" carries the highest and immediate priority.

Required Laboratory Data

Prothrombin time, partial thromboplastin time, and platelet count are desirable but may not be available because of the often emergent nature of this procedure.

PROCEDURE

1. The neck should be exposed and quickly examined, noting the thyroid and cricoid cartilages and the cricothyroid membrane. The anatomic landmarks usually are well defined and constant. The thyroid cartilage ("Adam's apple") is a large structure with a "V"-shaped notch in the midline at its superior aspect. Immediately below the thyroid cartilage is the cricoid ring, which is a complete circular ring denoting the

narrowest part of the airway. The space between the cricoid ring and the inferior aspect of the thyroid cartilage represents the cricothyroid membrane and is the site for airway access (Fig 19–1).

2. With proper immobilization of the patient's head, quickly cleanse the anterior neck with iodophor solution. Position a fenestrated drape over the neck, leaving the thyroid and cricoid cartilages visible.

3. Inject local anesthetic (approximately 2 to 3 mL of 1% lidocaine) into the cricoid area. Be careful to avoid obscuring the anatomy by injection of too large of volume of solution. In comatose patients, adminis-

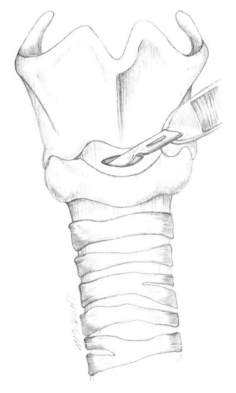

FIG. 19–1.
To enter the airway, make a transverse incision in the cricothyroid membrane.

tration of local anesthetic may be omitted.

4. Stand on the patient's right side and stabilize the thyroid cartilage by grasping it with the left hand.

5. With the scalpel (number 10 blade) in the right hand, incise transversely over the cricothyroid membrane for a distance of 3 to 4 cm, cutting through the dermis, platysma, and the cricothyroid membrane. (An acceptable alternative is to make a longitudinal incision in the midline over the cricothyroid area. A midline incision may bleed less than a transverse incision, but may provide less exposure than the transverse incision.)

6. Enter the airway through the cricothyroid membrane. (see Fig 19–1). Entry into the airway should be obvious, but could be obscured by bleeding, usually from the anterior jugular veins.

7. Enlarge and dilate the opening in the cricothyroid membrane by inserting a hemostat and spreading the tips with one hand (Fig 19–2). A tracheal spreader (Trousseau dilator) may also be used to enlarge the airway opening but is not mandatory.

8. Gently, but firmly, insert the endotracheal or tracheostomy tube into the trachea (Fig 19–3).

9. Inflate the cuff and connect the tube to a manual resuscitator bag, such as an Ambu bag. Auscultate for breath sounds over all lung fields and over the stomach.

10. With an endotracheal tube, right main stem bronchial intubation is common and should be anticipated.

11. Affix the airway to the skin with a silk suture.

12. Obtain a chest roentgenogram to verify appropriate placement of the artificial airway.

FOLLOW-UP

Immediately following placement of the airway, evaluate the adequacy of the patient's respiratory function. Carefully assess the airway on a daily basis; ensure that cuff inflation is maintained with appropriate cuff pressures. The appearance of the surrounding skin and the security of fixation should be noted. Gauze bandages may prevent pressure necrosis of the skin if applied in a padding fashion. Correction of all other physiologic derangements should proceed in a timely fashion.

Conversion of cricothyroidostomy to tracheostomy has been the standard recommendation in the past. There are few scientific data to support this practice. There is some evidence that a cricothyroidostomy may be the only airway necessary for long-term usage. Cri-

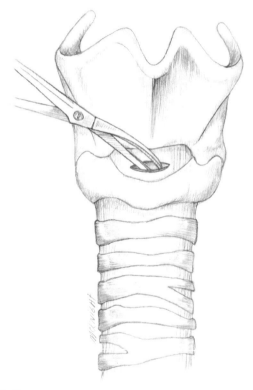

FIG. 19-2.
Enlarge the opening in the cricothyroid membrane by blunt dissection with the tips of a hemostat.

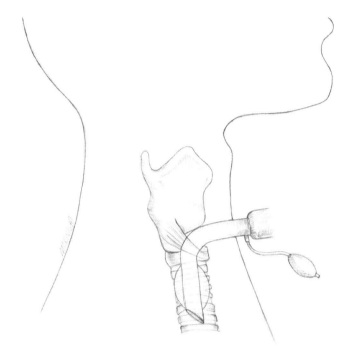

FIG. 19–3.
Tracheostomy tube passed through the cricothyroid membrane into the trachea.

cothyroidostomy has appeal to cardiac surgeons in patients with sternotomy incisions in that it separates the airway incision (contaminated) from the sternotomy (clean) and in theory lessens the risk of mediastinitis.

COMPLICATIONS

1. Local bleeding may be encountered but usually can be controlled easily after the airway is established.
2. Pneumomediastinum and subcutaneous emphysema may develop if dislodgement of the airway occurs.
3. Tracheoesophageal fistula and tracheoinnominate

artery fistula are two dreaded complications that, typically, occur later. These complications are potentially preventable by avoidance of excessive cuff pressures and early removal of rigid nasogastric tubes. Acute tracheoesophageal fistula may occur as a result of the posterior membranous trachea being violated at the time of insertion of the airway.

4. Tracheal stenosis is a late complication that occurs in a small but finite number of patients.

DOCUMENTATION

Write a note in the patient's chart that includes the following:

1. Indication for cricothyroidostomy.
2. Description of technique employed.
3. Complications, if any, encountered during procedure.
4. Size and type of airway inserted.
5. Findings of post-procedure chest roentgenogram performed to confirm tube position.

SUGGESTED READING

American College of Surgeons Committee of Trauma: *Advanced trauma life support course for physicians, instructor manual*, Chicago, 1985, American College of Surgeons, p 159.

Brantigan CO, Grow JB Sr: Subglottic stenosis after cricothyroidostomy, *Surgery* 91:217, 1982.

Brantigan CO, Grow JB Sr: Cricothyroidotomy: elective use in respiratory problems requiring tracheotomy, *J Thorac Cardiovasc Surg* 71(1):72, 1976.

Kress TD, Balasubramaniam S: Cricothyroidotomy, *Ann Emerg Med* 11:197, 1982.

McGill J et al: Cricothyrotomy in the emergency department, *Ann Emerg Med* 11:361, 1982.

Nunn DB et al: Trachea-innominate artery fistula following tracheostomy: successful repairs using an innominate vein graft, *Ann Thorac Surg* 20:698, 1975.

Romanita MC et al: Cricothyroidotomy—its healing and complications, *Surg Forum* 28:174, 1974.

20

Tracheostomy

Michael H. Albrink, M.D.

INTRODUCTION

Tracheostomy is a procedure that dates back 5,000 years, with references in ancient Egypt and India. There are references to surgical airways in the Old Testament and in Talmudic scripture. Surgical airway management was largely forgotten until this century. Early in this century, diphtheria epidemics led to performance of surgical airways. It is now a commonly performed procedure.

OBJECTIVE

To place and secure an artificial airway within the trachea by surgical incision in the neck.

Indications

1. Prolonged mechanical ventilation. Tracheostomy lessens the likelihood of injury to the larynx and vocal cords from prolonged translaryngeal intubation. The exact timing of performance of tracheostomy requires clinical judgement but is generally considered to be indicated between the 2nd and 3rd weeks of mechanical ventilation if weaning is not eminent.

2. Bronchial hygiene therapy. Patients with severe neurologic injury that are unable to handle pulmonary secretions.

3. Enhancement of patient comfort and increased ease of weaning from mechanical ventilation are purported benefits that are difficult to support by objective studies.

Contraindications

1. Hemodynamic instability and respiratory instability are contraindications to performance of tracheostomy until corrected.

2. Tracheostomy has some increased risk of mediastinitis if performed in early postoperative cardiac surgery (sternotomy) patients.

3. Uncontrolled coagulopathy is a relative contraindication, but this is a condition requiring clinical judgement.

PREPARATION

Careful scrutiny of the entire patient is necessary prior to performance of tracheostomy. Attention to possible reasons for respiratory insufficiency are to be noted and treated. If neurologic dysfunction is the indication for surgical airway, then careful search for a treatable cause is mandatory prior to any invasive procedure. Physical examination of the patient's neck and trachea is mandatory. Other wounds, intravenous devices, and other surgical procedures in this area should be noted. The presence of thyromegaly should be noted, as this condition can be difficult to manage in surgical tracheostomies.

At present, most tracheostomies are performed in the operating rooms. It has been shown that this procedure can be safely and efficiently performed at the patient's bedside in the setting of a closely monitored intensive care unit. Clinical judgement is needed to decide which patients are candidates for bedside procedures. Careful informed consent must be obtained from the patient and his/her family. The possibility of complications should be discussed with the patient and family, both for tracheostomy and prolonged translaryngeal intubation.

Equipment

Typical tracheostomy instrument sets come in prepared trays with usually more instruments than are needed.

1. Sterile drapes.
2. Sterile gowns.
3. Gloves and masks.
4. Iodophor solution.
5. Local anesthetic solution (lidocaine 1% to 2%).
6. Self-retaining retractors and "Army-Navy" retractors.
7. Scalpels.
8. Hemostats.
9. Tracheal spreaders.
10. Suture material.
11. A hook retractor.
12. Tracheostomy tubes: one tube of a size deemed appropriate for the patient, and one a size smaller.

Two essential components are

1. Electrocautery.
2. Good lighting.

Required Personnel

1. Of **greatest importance** is the presence of an anesthesiologist or intensivist to aid in removing the existing airway in a choreographed fashion. This person will also serve to re-establish the translaryngeal airway

should the surgical procedure become complicated and the airway lost.

2. Surgeon skilled in performance of a tracheostomy.
3. Surgical assistant.

Required Monitoring

1. Electrocardiogram.
2. Pulse oximeter.
3. Blood pressure, either by cuff or transduced arterial line.
4. End-tidal capnometry is helpful in diagnosis and management of many airway problems.
5. In patients with acute intracranial hypertension, intracranial pressure monitoring is advisable to alert to worsening of intracranial hypertension during the procedure.

Required Laboratory Data

1. Prothrombin time, partial thromboplastin time, and platelet count.
2. Arterial blood gas determinations are commonly used to document respiratory insufficiency.

PROCEDURE

1. Transfer the patient to the operating room and place supine on the table. Pay careful attention to monitoring of cardiopulmonary function during transport.
2. Slightly hyperextended the neck (only if the cervical spine is absolutely free of injury) and flex the table such that the patient's head is elevated about 30°. This will reduce venous pressure and lessen troublesome bleeding during the procedure.
3. Prepare the entire anterior neck, chin, mandibles, clavicles, and anterior chest wall with iodophor solution. Apply drapes in a manner that allows exposure for

both the operating surgeons to the neck and the anesthesiologist to the mouth.

4. Administer appropriate anesthesia to the patient. Local anesthesia, with or without supplemental intravenous sedation, or general anesthesia may be used.

5. Make a transverse skin incision approximately 1 to 2 cm above the clavicular heads. Extend the incision down through the platysma muscle in a similar transverse direction. Pay meticulous attention to hemostasis.

6. Once through the platysma, place a self-retaining retractor and dissect deeper in the midline in a cephalad-caudad direction. The midline offers the most hemostatic plane for access to the trachea.

7. Continue dissection in the midline between the strap muscles of the neck and replace the self-retaining retractor in a progressively deeper fashion.

8. It is wise to palpate the trachea frequently, to be sure that the dissection is directly in the midline. The most frequently encountered obstacles are the anterior jugular veins and the thyroid isthmus.

9. The anterior jugular veins course cephalad to caudad and commonly have a communicating "H" branch that usually will be found in the caudad portion of the wound. Tie off these veins and the communicating branch with silk ligatures and divide. This may prevent troublesome bleeding in the intensive care unit at later times.

10. Continue dissection down to the trachea (Fig 20–1). Exposure of the trachea should be relatively easy, with a noted exception being the isthmus of the thyroid. If the isthmus is encountered, displace with a gauze sponge in either a cephalad or caudad fashion to expose the appropriate portion of trachea. If necessary, the thyroid isthmus may be divided between clamps with suture ligature.

11. Once the trachea is reached, bluntly dissect with scissors or cautery and expose the anterior one third. Place "salvage" sutures of 3-0 polypropylene in the lateral aspects of the trachea, either around or through the second or third tracheal ring (Fig 20–2). Placement

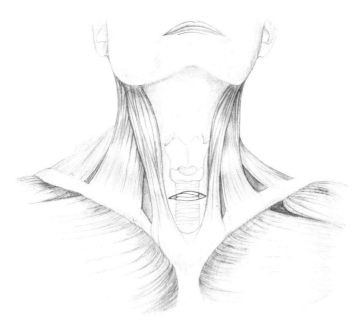

FIG 20–1.
Diagram showing exposure of the trachea through a transverse incision at the level of second to third tracheal rings.

of these important sutures often results in rupture of the balloon of the existing translaryngeal tube; this occurrence should be anticipated.

12. Prior to opening the trachea, check the tracheostomy tube and test the balloon. A tracheal spreader should be readily at hand; a tracheal hook retractor may be needed in elderly patients with kyphotic anatomy. Cervical and thoracic kyphosis often results in the trachea being well down in the mediastinum. A hook retractor is useful to pull up the trachea into the neck.

13. Before opening the trachea, alert the anesthesiologist or intensivist to prepare to remove the translaryngeal airway.

14. While tracheal incisions resembling all letters of the alphabet have been recommended, a longitudinal midline incision in the trachea is preferred. Make a longitudinal incision between the salvage sutures at the

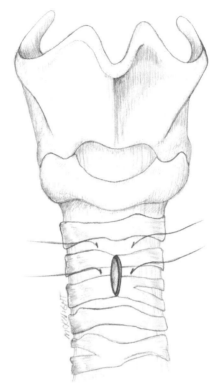

FIG 20–2.
Diagram showing the vertical incision in the trachea and the location of the salvage sutures.

level of the second and third tracheal rings (see Fig 20–2). There is always a minor amount of bleeding from the newly incised trachea; control this bleeding with cautery.

15. Once the trachea is opened, have the anesthesiologist slowly withdraw the existing endotracheal tube under direct guidance and vision of the surgeon—but not completely out of the larynx. When the tracheostomy tube is reliably placed, the anesthesiologist can remove the endotracheal tube completely.

16. Firmly introduce the tracheostomy tube into the tracheal opening, using the salvage sutures as traction

devices. Once the tube is in place, inflate the cuff and connect the tracheostomy to a device that enables ventilation with delivery of an appropriate oxygen concentration (for example, a manual resuscitator bag) (Fig 20–3). Confirmation of appropriate placement of the tracheostomy tube should be performed by auscultation by the anesthesiologist or intensivist, by observation of the pulse oximeter reading, and by noting end-tidal carbon dioxide tension (Pco_2) values.

17. If any question exists about the placement of the tracheostomy tube, remove the tube and reinsert the existing translaryngeal airway to ensure ventilation.

18. Repeat the steps outlined in 16 and 17 until suc-

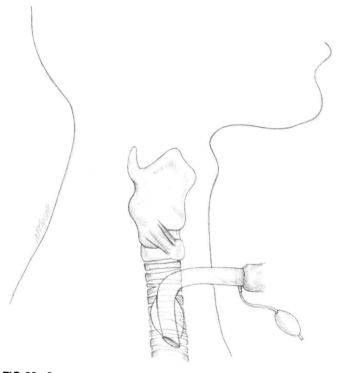

FIG 20–3.
Diagram showing the tracheostomy tube in the trachea with the tube cuff inflated.

cessful placement is ensured. Once intratracheal placement is secured, anchor the tracheostomy tube to the skin of the neck with several 3-0 polypropylene or nylon sutures. In addition, the tracheostomy tube should be anchored with umbilical tape placed around the patient's neck; umbilical tape around the neck should not be the sole source of fixation for the tracheostomy tube.

19. Once the procedure is completed, reconnect the patient to the ventilator and verify adequacy of ventilatory support. If ventilation is adequate, the patient may be returned to an intensive care unit.

FOLLOW-UP

1. Obtain a chest roentgenogram after the procedure to ensure proper placement of the tracheostomy tube and to rule out a pneumothorax.

2. Nursing personnel should inspect the tracheostomy site each shift. A physician should examine the site on a daily basis.

3. To avoid pressure necrosis of the surrounding skin under the collar of the tracheostomy tube, gauze bandages can be inserted as padding.

4. A routine schedule for changing tracheostomy tubes is probably not necessary, unless the tube (or more often the cuff) is not functioning properly.

COMPLICATIONS

It should be noted that in spite of perfect care, complications of tracheostomy are unavoidable in a certain small percentage of patients. There are many complications of tracheostomy including the following.

1. Tracheal stenosis.
2. Bleeding.
3. Hemorrhage.
4. Pneumothorax.

5. Air embolism.

6. Subcutaneous emphysema.

7. Two rare, though disastrous, complications of tracheostomy are tracheo-esophageal fistula and tracheo-innominate artery fistula. The incidence of these two complications, fortunately, has decreased with modern tracheostomy tubes that employ low-pressure, high-volume cuffs.

DOCUMENTATION

A progress note documenting the indication for the procedure should be placed prior to the procedure. The procedure should be documented after its performance by a brief progress note and a dictated operative note. Results of the postoperative chest roentgenogram also should be noted in the progress notes.

SUGGESTED READING

Grenvik A et al: Prolonged intubation for airway management in the intensive care unit. In Simmons RL, Udekwu AO, editors: *Debates in clinical surgery*, St Louis, 1991, Mosby–Year Book.

Hefner JE: Tracheal intubation in mechanically ventilated patients, *Clin Chest Med* 9:23, 1988.

Kirchner JC et al: Prolonged intubation vs. tracheotomy: complications, practical and psychological considerations, *Laryngoscope* 98:1165, 1988.

Stock MC et al: Peri-operative complications of elective tracheostomy in critically ill patients, *Crit Care Med* 14:861, 1986.

21

Tube Thoracostomy

Joan M. Christie, M.D
Michael H. Albrink, M.D.

INTRODUCTION

Normally, there is no space between the chest wall and lung. The pleural space can only be observed when air, blood, exudate, transudate, or chyle accumulate between visceral and parietal pleural surfaces.

Pleural fluid may impair pulmonary function by restricting ipsilateral lung function, leading to decreased lung compliance and hypoxemia. If a large volume of fluid accumulates in the pleural space, the pressure within the pleural space may rise, compromising both ipsilateral and contralateral lung and cardiac function. Accumulation of gas in the pleural space (pneumothorax) can lead to a rising intrapleural pressure (tension pneumothorax), particularly in patients receiving positive airway pressure. A tension pneumothorax markedly restricts lung function; impairs cardiac function; and, if uncorrected, rapidly leads to cardiopulmonary decompensation and arrest. Tube thoracostomy is indicated when the patient has respiratory or cardiac embarrassment secondary to air or fluid in the pleural space.

OBJECTIVE

To decompress the pleural space by insertion of a tube through the chest wall into the pleural space, a procedure termed tube thoracostomy.

Indications

Absolute indications include

1. Tension pneumothorax.
2. Empyema.

Relative indications include

1. Pneumothorax without tension.
2. Hemothorax.
3. Hydrothorax.
4. Any combination of these indications.

Contraindications

Infection at the site of proposed tube insertion.

PREPARATION

Establish the diagnosis of pleural fluid or gas by physical examination, confirmed by a chest roentgenogram. Ideally, the patient should be receiving additional oxygen to breathe.

Equipment

1. Mask, gown, gloves, sterile drapes.
2. Iodophor solution for skin preparation.
3. Sponges.
4. Local anesthetic solution, lidocaine 1%.
5. Syringe, 10 mL.
6. Hypodermic needle, 20 gauge.

7. Scalpel.

8. Hemostat or comparable instrument for blunt dissection.

9. Thoracostomy tube. Several varieties of plastic disposable thoracostomy tubes are available. The tube should have a radiopaque line and have more than six holes in the distal end. Additional holes can be cut on most tubes prior to insertion. Small tubes (24 F) tend to obstruct after placement and may require a trocar stylet for insertion. Trocar placement is not recommended, and many complications have occurred as a result of the use of a trocar. Large chest tubes (32 to 35 F) with radiopaque markers are preferred for most surgical and trauma patients.

10. Water-seal drainage collection apparatus. The simplest collection device for a thoracostomy tube is a gravity water seal drainage bottle (see "Procedure," item 13). Any fluid or gas in the pleural space exerting a pressure of more than 3 cm H_2O will drain into the bottle. Most contemporary commercial collection devices use a two-bottle principle that permits both gravity drainage and suction evacuation of the pleural space.

11. Suture material, sterile dressing, tape.

12. Specimen containers for appropriate culture, cytology, and laboratory procedures on any fluid drained from the pleural space. Procedures that may be performed include Gram stain, tuberculosis screening, fungal smears; culture of aerobic and anaerobic bacteria and fungus; cytologic studies; and assessments of protein, glucose, pH, lactic dehydrogenase, and amylase.

Required Monitoring

1. Continuous electrocardiography.

2. Pulse oximetry.

3. Blood pressure, either by continuous measurement through an indwelling arterial line or intermittently with a blood pressure cuff.

Required Laboratory Data

1. Arterial blood gas analysis.
2. Chest roentgenogram confirming diagnosis of pleural fluid or gas. If the clinical picture suggests a tension pneumothorax and the patient's cardiopulmonary function is unstable, omit the chest roentgenogram.

PROCEDURE

1. Introduce yourself to the patient and explain why and what you are about to do.
2. Obtain informed written consent. In an emergency situation, such as tension pneumothorax with decompensation of cardiopulmonary function, consent can be omitted because, in this circumstance, tube thoracostomy is a life-saving procedure.
3. Wash hands thoroughly and don sterile gloves and gown.
4. Prepare a 10-mL syringe with 1% lidocaine and a 20-gauge needle.
5. Ensure that the 32 to 35 F chest tube, water-seal drainage collection device, suture material, sterile dressing, and tape are on hand.
6. Place the patient supine, with the side for tube insertion uppermost. Support the patient's arm with a cushion above the head.
7. Identify the tube insertion site on the chest wall. The appropriate site for a thoracostomy tube depends on the substance distending the pleural space. In a supine patient, fluid initially collects posteriorly and inferiorly. In contrast, air rises to occupy an anterior and superior position in the hemithorax. Thus, thoracostomy tubes for pneumothorax are often positioned in the second intercostal space in the midclavicular line. In trauma patients, air and blood or other fluids frequently accumulate in the pleural space. Postero-superior thoracostomy tubes eliminate both air and fluid

and should be satisfactory in most clinical situations. Thus in traumatic or surgical patients, thoracostomy tubes frequently are placed in the fifth or sixth interspace in the midaxillary line, directed posteriorly and superiorly. More anterior insertion sites carry the risk of subdiaphragmatic tube placement.

Locate the sixth intercostal space in the midaxillary line. This position avoids major nerves and overlying muscle (Fig 21–1,A)

8. Cleanse the area with iodophor solution.

9. Anesthetize the insertion site. Raise a skin weal with 1% lidocaine, and then deposit 5 to 10 mL of local anesthetic solution in the chest wall. Local anesthesia is usually sufficient. However, intravenous sedation may be necessary for some patients. Administer sedation by careful intravenous titration to the desired endpoint to avoid depression of respiratory efforts.

10. Make a 2- to 3-cm incision midway between the ribs through the skin and superficial intercostal muscles (Fig 21–1,B). Avoid the neurovascular bundle which lies in the intercostal groove on the inferior surface of the rib.

11. Separate the tissues down to the pleural space by blunt dissection with a hemostat. Puncture of the parietal pleura may require considerable pressure to be exerted with the tip of the hemostat. Gently insert your index finger into the chest to open the space and clear away pleural adhesions (Fig 21–1,C).

12. Insert a 32 to 35 F thoracostomy tube through the opening in the chest wall (Fig 21-1,D). Make sure that all thoracostomy tube drainage holes are within the pleural cavity and not outside or within the skin.

13. Clamp the thoracostomy tube and connect it to a water seal drainage system (Fig 21-1,E). Remember that in a patient with a pneumothorax there is the risk of a tension pneumothorax developing while the tube is clamped; keep the clamp time as short as possible.

14. Remove the clamp from the thoracostomy tube. If air has collected in the pleural space, bubbles will be seen in the collection apparatus.

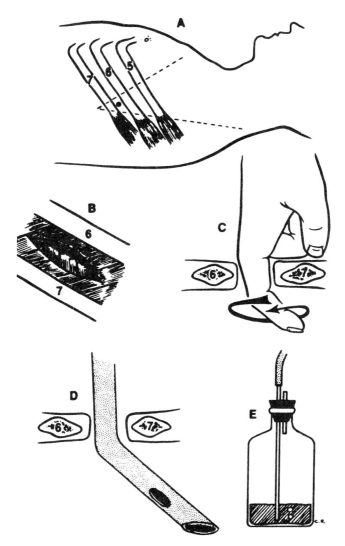

FIG 21-1.
Tube thoracostomy. **A,** the patient is positioned supine and the sixth intercostal space in the midaxillary line is identified. **B,** an incision is made in the middle of the interspace through the intercostal muscles and the opening into the pleural space completed with blunt dissection. **C,** blood and pleural adhesions are cleared by a circular motion of a finger inserted through the opening. **D,** the chest tube is inserted into the pleural space. **E,** the thoracostomy tube is connected to a water seal drainage system. (From Condon RE, Nyhus LM: *Manual of surgical therapeutics,* ed 7, Boston, 1988, Little Brown, p 387. Used by permission.)

15. Pleural fluid, if present, should drain easily from the thoracostomy tube into the drainage system. The water seal apparatus must be kept below the level of the patient's chest at all times.

16. Turn the suction on if large amounts of pleural fluid are to be evacuated. Suction is not needed for a simple pneumothorax unless the lung fails to expand.

17. Suture the wound and secure the thoracostomy tube to the skin. Some surgeons prefer to tunnel the thoracostomy tube subcutaneously for a short distance, a practice that is seldom necessary in adult patients.

18. Obtain a chest roentgenogram after thoracostomy tube insertion.

FOLLOW-UP

1. Check the chest roentgenogram for tube position.

2. Obtain arterial blood gas analysis to verify adequacy of ventilation and oxygenation.

3. Check the amount and nature of any drainage from the thoracostomy tube daily.

4. Inspect the insertion site daily for evidence of infection.

5. If clinically indicated, collect pleural fluid samples for laboratory analysis.

6. Consider removal of the thoracostomy tube when drainage ceases and examination of the patient, clinically and with roentgenography, shows the lung to be fully expanded and the pleural space free of fluid and gas.

COMPLICATIONS

1. Thoracostomy tube malposition.
   a. Tube is not in the chest (for example, in the liver, or subcutaneous space).
   b. Tube is in the chest but too high or too low to be effective. The thoracostomy tube should be

repositioned to optimize drainage of air (anterosuperior position) or fluid (place low in the sixth intercostal space in the midaxillary line).
   c. Tube is in the chest but not in the pleural space, (for example, in the pulmonary parenchyma).
2. Empyema or wound infection at insertion site.
3. Blockage of the thoracostomy tube by blood or fibrin clot.
4. Application of excessive suction on the thoracostomy tube may exsanguinate a patient with a hemothorax that is actively bleeding or may produce respiratory embarrassment. Suction may be increased to high levels if a patient has a persistent air leak and the lung does not re-expand.

DOCUMENTATION

Write and sign a tube thoracostomy note in the progress notes of the patient's chart. Include the following:

1. Whether or not informed consent was obtained from the patient or guardian.
2. The indication for the procedure.
3. The dose of local anesthetic administered.
4. The site of tube insertion.
5. The size of thoracostomy tube used.
6. The volume and appearance of any fluid obtained.
7. A description of the efficacy of the water seal drainage apparatus, including the following.
   a. Gas bubbling if the patient has a pneumothorax and the water level in the drainage system fluctuates with respirations.
   b. The amount of suction applied to the device, if applicable.
   c. The rate of accumulation of fluid in the drainage chamber.
8. Laboratory tests ordered for fluid analysis.

9. The outcome of the procedure and any complications that occurred during the procedure.
10. The findings of the follow-up chest roentgenogram and arterial blood gas analysis.
11. The condition of the patient at the end of the procedure.

SUGGESTED READING

Bryant LR, Morgan CV: Chest wall, pleura, lung and mediastinum. In Schwartz SI et al, editors: *Principles of surgery,* ed 4, New York, 1983, McGraw Hill.

Moore FA, Moore EE: Trauma resuscitation, In Wilmore DW et al, editors: *The American College of Surgeons care of the surgical patient,* volume I, *Critical care, New York,* 1991, Scientific American, p 27.

22

Conventional Mechanical Ventilatory Support

Roy D. Cane, M.B.B.Ch., F.F.A.(S.A.)

INTRODUCTION

Mechanical ventilatory support is associated with significant disruption of normal cardiopulmonary function and is not without risks. Therefore, a safe, consistent technique for committing a patient to mechanical ventilatory support is essential. Although the following protocol is by no means the only way to initiate mechanical ventilatory support, it can be applied fairly universally, is based on sound knowledge of cardiopulmonary function and ventilator technology, and has been used safely in a large number of critically ill patients.

Background Information

Modern ventilators function in several different modes (Table 22–1). Ventilator modes can be divided into two major categories on the basis of delivered vol-

TABLE 22–1.

Description of Ventilator Modes

Mode	Interaction Between Ventilator and Patient
Control mode ventilation	Patient does not participate in any phase of breathing cycle
Assist/control mode ventilation	Ventilator breath initiated by patient's inspiratory effort.
	Ventilator rate set by patient, if patient's respiratory rate is greater than the preset CMV rate
Intermittent mandatory ventilation	Patient breathes spontaneously by means of a continuous flow circuit in between ventilator breaths delivered at preset intervals
Synchronized intermittent mandatory ventilation	Patient breathes spontaneously by means of a demand flow circuit in between ventilator breaths delivered at preset intervals in synchrony with patient's inspiratory effort
Pressure support ventilation	Patient's inspiratory effort determines the rate.
	Ventilator maintains preset inspiratory pressure.
	Inspiration ends when patient's inspiratory flow falls below preset minimal value.

ume/breath. Volume-preset modes [control mode ventilation (CMV), assist/control mode ventilation (A/CMV), intermittent mandatory ventilation (IMV), and synchronized IMV (SIMV)] deliver a preset tidal volume (V_T) unless specified safety limits are exceeded, whereas the volume-variable mode [pressure support ventilation (PS)] delivers unspecified tidal volumes determined by the interaction of preset ventilator and patient factors. The modes define the relationship between the patient and ventilator with respect to the manner in which inspiration is initiated, regulated, and powered (Table 22–2). Choice of a particular mode should be based on consideration of patient and ventilator factors, to determine the best approach.

Ventilators may be set to provide full or partial ventilatory support. Full ventilatory support (FVS), defined as provision of positive pressure ventilation (PPV) in a

TABLE 22–2.

Physical Characteristics Associated With Initiation, Limitation, and Cycling of the Inspiratory Phase of Mechanical Breath for Each Ventilator Mode*

Ventilator Mode†	Initiated	Limited	Cycled
CMV	Time	Volume	Volume/time
A/CMV	Pressure	Volume	Volume/time
IMV	Time	Volume	Volume/time
SIMV	Pressure	Volume	Volume/time
PS	Pressure	Pressure	Flow

*From Shapiro BA et al: Modes of positive pressure ventilation. In *Clinical application of respiratory care*, ed 4, St Louis, 1991, Mosby–Year Book, p 304. Used by permission.

†CMV = control mode ventilation; A/CMV = assist/CMV; IMV = intermittent mandatory ventilation; SIMV = synchronized IMV; PS = pressure support ventilation. For a discussion of ventilator modes see the text (Background Information) and Table 22–1.

manner that ensures that the patient is **not required** to contribute to the physiologic alveolar ventilation, can be provided by any of the ventilator modes. Partial ventilatory support (PVS), defined as provision of PPV in a manner that **obligates** the patient to provide some of the physiologic alveolar ventilation, can be provided only by the IMV, SIMV, and PS modes. Theoretic advantages of PVS over FVS include

1. More stable cardiovascular function.
2. Better distribution of ventilation.
3. Less disuse atrophy of ventilatory muscles.
4. Less sedation required.

The advantages of PVS make it the preferred method for prolonged ventilatory support (more than 24 hours) of the patient with stable cardiovascular and central nervous system function, and during weaning from PPV.

OBJECTIVE

Safe initiation and maintenance of mechanical ventilatory support of an acute critically ill patient.

Indications

1. Apnea.
2. Acute ventilatory failure.
3. Impending ventilatory failure.
    a. To relieve work of breathing.
    b. To relieve work of the heart.
4. Anticipated ventilatory failure.
    a. Elective postoperative ventilatory support.

Contraindications

1. Absolute: none.
2. Relative:
    a. "Do not resuscitate" status.
    b. Ventilatory failure secondary to irreversible cardiopulmonary disease.

Specific Indications for Full Ventilatory Support

1. Initial ventilatory support.
    a. Patients with unstable heart function.
    b. Need to assume the work of breathing completely.
2. Prolonged ventilatory support.
    a. Chronic apnea.
    b. Utilization of ventilator circuit deadspace tubing to achieve eucapnia.
    c. Intolerance of partial ventilatory support.

Usual ventilator settings for volume-preset modes are VTs between 10 and 20 mL/kg, delivered within an inspiratory time of 0.5 to 1.5 seconds at rates of eight or more breaths per minute for FVS and seven or fewer per minute for PVS. Settings for the volume-variable mode are determined by titrating the level of positive inspiratory pressure to achieve a tidal volume of 10 to 20 mL/kg for FVS or a clinically acceptable respiratory rate for PVS. All modes of ventilatory support can be used in conjunction with positive end-expiratory pressure (PEEP) or continuous positive airway pressure (CPAP) (see Chapter 24). Positive pressure ventilation

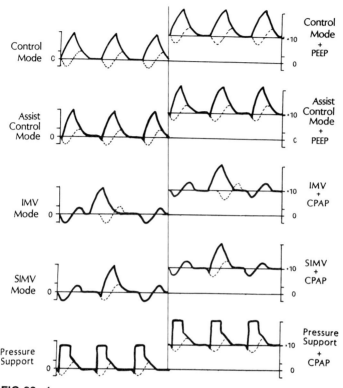

FIG 22–1.
Airway pressure tracings for commonly employed modes of ventilation. *Left hand tracings* depict ventilation without PEEP. *Right hand tracings* show ventilation with addition of $+10$ cm H_2O PEEP or CPAP. (Modified from Shapiro BA et al: Modes of positive pressure ventilation. In *Clinical application of respiratory care*, ed 4, St Louis, Mosby–Year Book, 1991. Used by permission.)

with PEEP or CPAP is associated with a potentially higher incidence of disadvantageous physiologic effects and complications. The airway pressure patterns of the different modes with and without PEEP/CPAP are shown in Figure 22–1.

PREPARATION

Evaluate the patient with respect to indications for FVS or PVS. For patients without specific indications for FVS, provide initial support with FVS for the first 12 to 24 hours. Thereafter, switch to PVS and titrate mechanical ventilatory support to the minimum associated with stable cardiopulmonary function. Although the pressure support mode can provide FVS, using it for FVS offers no apparent clinical advantages. Therefore, the pressure support mode is recommended for PVS only.

Equipment

1. Manual ventilator with appropriate oxygen source and fraction of inspired oxygen (FIO_2).
2. Ventilator.
3. Pulse oximeter.

Required Monitoring

1. Electrocardiography (EKG).
2. Blood pressure (BP) through an arterial line or BP cuff.
3. Pulse oximetry.
4. Capnography (optional).
5. Transcutaneous monitoring of carbon dioxide ($P_{tc}CO_2$) (optional).

Required Laboratory Data

1. Arterial blood gas analysis.
2. Chest roentgenogram confirming endotracheal (ET) tube placement.

PROCEDURE

Committing a patient to a ventilator is a staged procedure.

1. Initial FVS.
   a. Patient preparation.

    b. Connection to ventilator.
    c. Verification of adequacy of mechanical ventilatory support.
2. Prolonged Support with PVS.
    a. Volume-preset modes (IMV, SIMV).
    b. Volume-variable mode (PS).

Initial Full Ventilatory Support

1. Patient Preparation
    a. Introduce yourself to the patient and explain why ventilatory support is necessary. Reassure the patient that you will be there throughout the initial period of ventilator commitment, that the ventilator will help him/her breathe, and that he/she will receive appropriate sedation (see Chapter 13).
    b. Establish an artificial airway and manually support ventilation. Provision of PPV in the acute critically ill adult requires an artificial airway to ensure a stable connection to the ventilator circuit and to minimize gastric distention. Place a naso-tracheal or ET tube. Verify the ET tube position (see Chapter 18).
    c. Following intubation, assist the patient's ventilatory efforts manually with a self-inflating bag with a one-way valve system (for example, Ambu bag) connected to appropriate oxygen source. Manual ventilation has the following advantages.
       (1) It is immediately available.
       (2) It can easily be varied from moment to moment.
       (3) It is relatively simple.
       (4) It provides continuous feedback regarding the system compliance and resistance, and the patient's spontaneous ventilatory efforts. Moreover, it allows the flexibility of trial and error in attempts to establish the ideal ventilatory pattern.

d. Stabilize the cardiovascular system.
Cardiovascular instability, characterized by
hypotension and/or cardiac arrhythmias
secondary to decreased venous return and
sympathetic tone, is not uncommon following
initiation of PPV. If cardiovascular instability
develops following initiation of PPV with the
manual ventilator, elevate the patient's feet 20°
to 30° from horizontal, administer intravenous
fluids (0.9N saline), and manually ventilate in
synchrony with the patient's spontaneous efforts,
allowing long expiratory periods (longer than
double the inspiratory time). If these measures
are not effective, consider the use of inotropic
support.

e. Evaluate the patient's status and establish
monitors. Ideally, the patient's baseline vital
signs and arterial blood gases (ABG) will have
been determined prior to initiation of ventilatory
support. If time was insufficient to establish the
necessary monitors (EKG, BP, pulse oximeter)
before, do so now. Evaluate the patient's
cardiovascular status pulse oximetry (Sp_{O_2}) and
end-tidal CO_2 tension/transcutaneous carbon
dioxide tension ($P_{ET}CO_2/P_{tc}CO_2$, if available); obtain
ABG evaluation.

f. Select the ventilatory pattern. Because PPV is
associated with an increase in deadspace
ventilation, supranormal minute ventilation is
required. Ventilator settings that deliver 8 L/min
provide a reasonable starting point. Large
mechanical (V_T)s of 12 to 15 ML/kg ideal body
weight are recommended. If the patient's disease
state is likely to have resulted in significantly
reduced lung compliance, V_Ts of 10 to 12 mL/kg
are reasonable. Select a ventilator rate that,
when multiplied by the selected V_T will give a
minute ventilation of approximately 8 L/min.

g. Establish the chosen ventilatory pattern. The
patient's spontaneous ventilatory efforts should

be initially augmented by manual ventilation. Usually, patients will gradually relax and accept a slower, deeper pattern of ventilation. Duplicate the chosen ventilatory pattern with manual ventilation. If the patient is stable and accepts the pattern of ventilation, he/she is ready for commitment to the ventilator. If the pattern is not tolerated by the patient, adjust the pattern or consider use of sedation or muscle relaxants.

2. Connect the patient to the ventilator. Once the patient has been prepared, and the mechanical ventilator appropriately set and tested, connect the patient to the ventilator. Immediately following connection of the patient and for the subsequent 15 minutes, a clinician must closely monitor the patient's cardiopulmonary status and ventilator function.

3. Verification of adequacy of ventilatory support. The goal of ventilatory support is provision of sufficient alveolar ventilation to maintain cardiopulmonary homeostasis. The only absolutely reliable measure of the adequacy of alveolar ventilation is measurement of the arterial tension of carbon dioxide ($Paco_2$). Therefore, obtain an ABG evaluation after 15 minutes to verify that the appropriate support of ventilation has been achieved. A transcutaneous CO_2 tension ($P_{tc}co_2$) gives a reliable reflection of the $Paco_2$ provided that skin perfusion is within reasonably normal limits. Measurement of the $P_{ET}co_2$ is only reliable as a reflector of the $Paco_2$ if the patient has normal lung function and a normal cardiac output.

   a. If ABG or $P_{tc}co_2$ reveal hyperventilation, decrease ventilation by reducing the ventilator rate or V_T. In most circumstances, reduce the ventilator rate as a primary step; consider reduction of V_T if the pattern of ventilation has resulted in a high peak airway pressure (over 45 cm H_2O). Remember, high ventilator rates are associated with greater amounts of deadspace

INTERMITTENT MANDATORY VENTILATION

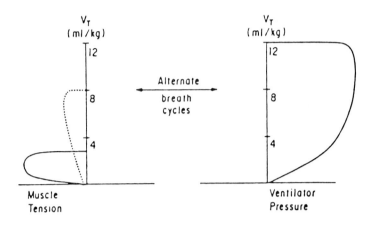

PRESSURE SUPPORT VENTILATION

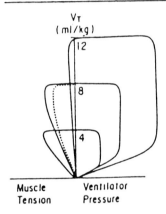

FIG 22–2.
Schematic diagrams representing the quantity and the characteristics of the patient's and ventilator's contributions to the work of breathing during various modes of mechanical ventilatory support. In each panel, work per tidal breath is depicted as the area inscribed by the pressure-volume relationships during that breath. Spontaneous breaths are depicted with *left-ward-directed* muscle tension or intramuscular pressure. Ventilator breaths are depicted with *rightward-directed* airway pressure. The *dashed line* represents a normal pressure-volume relationship. **Top,** intermittent mandatory ventilation is depicted. This approach allows patients to work in between mandatory ventilator breaths. Patient work quantity is thus controlled by the number of mandatory breaths given while work characteristics are again fixed in a higher than normal pressure/volume

ventilation and greater potential for creation of intrinsic PEEP. (See Complications.)

b. If ABG or $P_{tc}CO_2$ values reveal hypoventilation, increase the ventilation by increasing the V_T in 100- to 200-mL increments. If the peak airway pressure is high, increase ventilation by increasing the ventilator rate.

Prolonged Support With Partial Ventilatory Support

Evaluate the patient to determine that no specific indications for FVS are evident. Patients should have had stable vital signs and ABG or Spo_2 for the preceding several hours before a switch to PVS is attempted.

Choose either a volume-preset or volume-variable mode. There are no data supporting the advantage of either volume-preset or volume-variable modes for the provision of PVS. Pressure support ventilation has theoretical advantages over IMV/SIMV. Because PS assists every breath, the level of support will increase proportionately if a rising minute ventilatory demand secondary to increased CO_2 production results in a higher respiratory rate; IMV/SIMV provides a *fixed* contribution to the required minute ventilation that is independent of spontaneous respiratory rate. The high-volume, low-pressure spontaneous inspiratory work characteristics associated with PS are closer to the physiologic normal pattern than the low-volume, high-pressure, spontaneous inspiratory work characteristics associated with IMV/SIMV. The work characteristics of PS may have a beneficial effect on ventilatory muscle conditioning (Fig 22–2). Choice of mode is at present a matter of physician preference.

configuration. **Bottom,** pressure support ventilation is depicted. Patient work quantity is controlled by the level of pressure applied with every breath. Unlike volume-cycle ventilator modes, work characteristics are changed with pressure support ventilation to a more normal configuration. (From Kirby RR et al: Pressure support ventilation. In *Problems in critical care,* vol 4, *Positive pressure ventilation,* Philadelphia, JB Lippincott, p 227. Used by permission.)

1. Volume-preset modes (IMV, SIMV). Intermittent mandatory ventilation employs a circuit with a continuous gas flow for spontaneous breaths, whereas SIMV employs a circuit with a demand valve to provide a gas source for spontaneous breaths. The SIMV mode is associated with greater spontaneous inspiratory work (opening the demand valve) than is IMV. This difference in work is only significant in patients with minimal ventilatory reserve.

    a. Obtain baseline vital signs and ABG values.
    b. While closely monitoring the patient's ability to tolerate the spontaneous work of breathing, reduce IMV/SIMV rate in decrements of one to two machine breaths per minute. The patient's spontaneous respiratory rate is probably the most reliable reflector of tolerance of the work of breathing. Development of tachypnea, tachycardia, systolic hypertension, or complaints of dyspnea suggest an inadequate level of ventilatory support.
    c. Continue to reduce IMV/SIMV rate to the lowest level associated with stable vital signs and a spontaneous respiratory rate between 10 and 20 breaths per minute.
    d. After 15 to 30 minutes on a given level of IMV/SIMV, repeat ABG study to verify the adequacy of alveolar ventilation.

2. Volume-variable mode (PS). Pressure support ventilation can be provided in conjunction with IMV/SIMV but not with CMV or A/CMV. To ensure a smooth transition from FVS to PVS with PS, it is advisable to have the ventilator set in the IMV or SIMV mode prior to initiating the change to PS.

    a. Set ventilator to IMV/SIMV plus PS.
    b. Set a PS level of approximately half the peak inspiratory pressure seen with an IMV/SIMV breath.
    c. Obtain baseline vital signs and ABG values.
    d. Reduce the IMV/SIMV rate to four machine

breaths per minute and observe the patient's spontaneous respiratory rate for 10 to 15 minutes.

Note: If the patient's spontaneous respiratory rate is greater than 20 breaths per minute after this step (that is, on IMV/SIMV of four breaths per minute plus PS), re-evaluate the patient with respect to suitability for PSV.

e. Provided the patient's respiratory rate is less than 20 breaths per minute, discontinue the IMV/SIMV. At this point, the patient will be supported only with PS.

f. Make further adjustments in PS level, depending on the patient's spontaneous respiratory rate. If the patient's respiratory rate is still less than 20 breaths per minute, decrease the PS level in 3- to 5-cm-H_2O decrements until the respiratory rate is between 10 to 20 breaths per minute and vital signs remain stable. This pressure represents an appropriate level of PS for PVS.

g. If the patient's respiratory rate is greater than 20 breaths per minute, increase the PS level by 3- to 5-cm-H_2O increments until his/her respiratory rate is between 10 to 20 breaths per minute.

h. After 15 to 30 minutes, obtain ABG or $P_{tc}co_2$ measurements to verify adequacy of alveolar ventilation.

During ventilatory support, whenever patient instability or mechanical problems arise, the patient must be disconnected from the ventilator and manually ventilated.

FOLLOW-UP

1. Repeat ABG measurements as necessary; the required frequency depends on the stability of the patient's condition. Remember that re-evaluating the adequacy of ventilatory support after any change in

ventilator settings or patient condition is mandatory. All patients on FVS and many patients on PVS cannot increase their minute ventilation in response to an increase in CO_2 production (for example, following initiation of, or increase in, nutritional support). Thus, ABG measurements should be obtained whenever a change in CO_2 production is suspected and also checked 20 to 30 minutes after any change in ventilator settings.

2. Obtain a daily chest roentgenogram to check for development of complications: in particular, pneumonia, atelectasis, and barotrauma.

3. Evaluate the need for continued ventilatory support daily. Mechanical ventilatory support is hazardous; therefore, timely discontinuance of ventilatory support is every bit as important as timely initiation of ventilatory support.

COMPLICATIONS

1. *Physiologic disadvantages of PPV.*
   a. Positive airway pressure produces an increase in intrathoracic pressures and right atrial pressure that result in a decrease in venous return to the right side of the heart.
   b. Higher alveolar pressures increase the distribution of pulmonary perfusion to dependent regions of lung, resulting in an increase in number of ventilated, but poorly perfused, alveoli.
   c. Positive pressure ventilation tends to result in greater distribution of ventilation to those areas of lung with highest compliance and lowest airway resistance (the nondependent lung).
      The major physiologic disadvantage of PPV, therefore, is an increase in deadspace ventilation.
2. *Complications.*
   a. Mechanical malfunction is always potentially present. If a mechanical problem occurs,

disconnect the patient from the ventilator and manually ventilate.

b. The condition in which a patient is out of phase with ventilator, commonly referred to as "bucking or fighting the ventilator," may be associated with either mechanical or patient factors. These include equipment malfunction, intolerance of the ventilator mode, endotracheal tube displacement, pain, hypoxemia, arrhythmias, hypercapnia, and acidosis.

c. Intrinsic PEEP. If exhalation is not completed before the next inspiration, end-expiratory pressure can rise above baseline level (so-called intrinsic PEEP). This problem may occur with ventilator settings of a rapid ventilator rate (usually above 15 breaths per minute) and large V_T or if the patient has a high expiratory airway resistance, for example in chronic obstructive pulmonary disease or asthma. Intrinsic PEEP has the potential to increase the onset of cardiovascular instability and development of barotrauma.

d. Cardiovascular instability, manifesting as hypotension and cardiac arrhythmias, is secondary to decreased venous return and sympathetic tone. The physiologic and psychologic stresses on the patient prior to provision of ventilatory support frequently result in sympathetic nervous system stimulation; increased catecholamine secretion; and, hence, venous constriction. Positive pressure ventilation ameliorates these stresses, leading to a reduction in sympathetic tone and resulting in a relative hypovolemia.

e. Barotrauma may manifest as subcutaneous emphysema, interstitial emphysema, pneumomediastinum, pneumothorax, pneumopericardium, or pneumoperitoneum. Barotrauma occurs in 7% to 10% of critically ill patients receiving PPV. Barotrauma occurs most commonly in patients with pre-existing lung disease and in those with a history of penetrating wounds of the thorax.

f. Infection and lobar or segmental atelectasis.

g. Gastrointestinal malfunction. Commonly, gastrointestinal bleeding is seen in ± 40% of patients on PPV for more than 3 days. Ileus and gastric dilatation may occur, particularly if the patient is receiving heavy sedation. Splanchnic blood flow may be decreased.

h. Renal malfunction. Positive pressure ventilation may result in sodium and water retention and decreased urine output secondary to changes in intrarenal blood flow and/or increased production of antidiuretic hormone.

i. Positive water balance may result from the renal changes in conjunction with the ventilator humidifier producing a net water gain by way of the respiratory tract.

j. Psychological trauma and dependence on mechanical ventilator may develop, although they are rare.

DOCUMENTATION

Write a note in the patient's chart that includes

1. Indication for institution of PPV.
2. Size and nature of airway.
3. Choice of ventilator mode.
4. Pre-PPV and post-PPV vital signs and ABG or P_{tcCO_2} and SpO_2 values.

At the time of initiation of PPV write, *Ventilator Orders,* which includes the following

1. Type of ventilator.
2. Ventilator mode.
3. Ventilator rate.

4. Exhaled V_T, in milliliters.
5. Fraction of inspired oxygen.
6. The PEEP/CPAP level, if needed.
7. Frequency of ABG monitoring and "Call Physician" parameters (for example, if the pH is less than 7.3 or exceeds 7.55; if CO_2 tension is less than 30 mm Hg or exceeds 55 mm Hg; and if the oxygen tension is less than 70 mm Hg or exceeds 100 mm Hg).

SUGGESTED READING

Kirby RR: Intermittent mandatory ventilation. In Perel A, Stock MC, editors: *Mechanical ventilatory support*, Baltimore, 1991, Williams & Wilkins, pp 101–116.

MacIntyre NR: Pressure support ventilation. In Perel A, Stock MC, editors: *Mechanical ventilatory support*, Baltimore, 1991, Williams & Wilkins, pp 129–136.

Marcy TW, Marini JJ: Controlled mechanical ventilation and assist/control ventilation. In Perel A, Stock MC, editors: *Mechanical ventilatory support*, Baltimore, 1991, Williams & Wilkins, pp 81–100.

Shapiro BA, Cane RD: Conventional mechanical ventilation. In Cane RD et al, editors: *Case studies in critical care medicine*, ed 2, St Louis, 1990, Mosby– Year Book, pp 52–81.

Stock MC, Perel A: Ventilatory support: temptations and pitfalls. In Perel A, Stock MC, editors: *Mechanical ventilatory support*, Baltimore, 1991, Williams & Wilkins, pp 177–286.

23

Discontinuing Mechanical Ventilatory Support

Roy D. Cane, M.B.B.Ch., F.F.A. (S.A.)

INTRODUCTION

Ventilator discontinuance may be achieved by one of two approaches:

1. Ventilatory challenge.
2. Gradual weaning.

Ventilatory Challenge

An adequate central nervous system stimulus, provided by the pH of the cerebrospinal fluid (CSF), is essential for maintaining spontaneous ventilation. Acute changes in arterial tension of carbon dioxide (Pco_2) are immediately reflected in the CSF and induce a change in CSF pH. A well-oxygenated, 70-kg person with a basal metabolic rate produces enough carbon dioxide in 1 minute to increase the Pco_2 of the blood 1 to 2 mm Hg, assuming no carbon dioxide is excreted by the lungs. The venous, alveolar, and arterial Pco_2 will equilibrate within the first minute of no ventilation, resulting in a 4- to 6-mm-Hg rise in arterial carbon dioxide tension ($Paco_2$). Theoretically, 5 minutes without ventilation should result in no more than a 15-mm-Hg rise in $Paco_2$. These predictable changes in CSF pH provide the basis for a safe and predictable approach to ventilator discontinuance in patients without pre-existing significant chronic cardiopulmonary disease—the ventilatory challenge.

Gradual Weaning

Discontinuing positive pressure ventilation (PPV) in patients with pre-existing significant chronic cardiopulmonary disease, or in those committed to PPV because of excessive work of breathing (WOB), is usually best achieved by a gradual decremental reduction in ventilatory support. Close monitoring of the patient's tolerance for the WOB after each decrement in ventilatory support is necessary. The majority of patients committed to PPV for appropriate, clear-cut indications and maintained with eucapnic ventilation can be taken off PPV by the ventilatory challenge technique.

OBJECTIVE

Safely discontinue mechanical ventilatory support of the critically ill patient.

Indications

Reversal or significant improvement of the disease process that necessitated mechanical ventilatory support.

Contraindications

1. Absence of intrinsic ventilatory drive.
2. Inadequate ventilatory muscle power or endurance.

PREPARATION

The decision to discontinue mechanical ventilatory support of a patient is a clinical judgment based largely upon clinical assessment of the patient. The important questions to be considered prior to discontinuance of PPV include the following.

1. Has the underlying disease that necessitated PPV been reversed or significantly improved? The clinical judgement that the underlying pathologic condition has resolved or significantly improved should immediately initiate evaluation of the patient's ventilatory reserve.

2. Does the patient have adequate cardiopulmonary reserves to assume the WOB?

3. Is the patient's cardiopulmonary function sufficient for adequate pulmonary gas exchange?

4. Are there any reversible factors that will increase the required WOB?

Assessment of Ventilatory Reserve

1. Spontaneous ventilatory function.
   a. The vital capacity (VC) is the largest breath that can be inspired. Normal tidal volumes (VT) are approximately 10% of the VC. Under circumstances of increased ventilatory demand a VT greater than 10% of the VC may be required. The greater the portion of the VC that is necessary for VT, the less will be the ability of the patient to increase VT to meet that demand. Thus, VC may be used as a clinical indicator of ventilatory reserve. The greater the portion of the VC that is used for VT, the greater is the WOB (Fig 23-1). Patients seldom tolerate the WOB associated with a VT that exceeds 30% to 40% of their VC. A VC of at least 15 mL/kg represents a reasonable minimum ventilatory reserve.

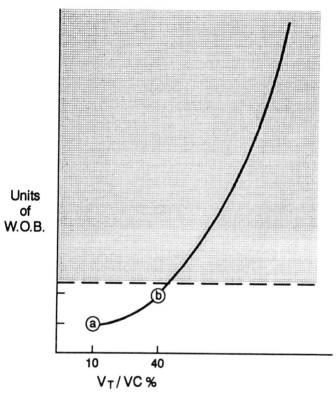

Units of W.O.B.

Ⓐ

Ⓑ

10   40

V_T/ VC %

FIG 23–1.
The work of breathing *(W.O.B.)* in relation to vital capacity *(VC).* Point *a* represents a V$_T$ of 500 mL with a VC of 5 L; point *b* represents a V$_T$ of 400 mL with a VC of 1 L. (From Acute respiratory failure. In Shapiro BA et al: *Clinical application of blood gases,* ed 4, St. Louis, 1989, Mosby–Year Book, p 259. Used by permission.)

b. A negative inspiratory force (NIF) of at least 20 cm H$_2$O in 20 seconds suggests that the patient should have a VC at least three times the predicted V$_T$.

c. Respiratory rate (RR). A regular pattern of breathing at less than 25 breaths per minute is desirable.

d. Tidal volumes are difficult to assess prior to the patient breathing spontaneously for a period of time. Initial V$_T$s of over 2 ml/kg are encouraging.

2. Cardiopulmonary Assessment.
   a. *Arterial blood gas (ABG).* Ideally the patient should show a normal acid-base balance, eucapnia, and normal arterial oxygen tension (Pa_{O_2}) with/without oxygen or positive end-expiratory pressure (PEEP) therapy. If $FI_{O_2} >$ 0.4, despite appropriate PEEP/continuous positive airway pressure (CPAP) therapy, is required to maintain a Pa_{O_2} of more than 60 mm Hg, reconsider whether the patient is ready for discontinuing ventilatory support. Remember that "normal" values for patients with chronic cardiopulmonary disease may be a Pa_{CO_2} greater than 45 mm Hg and a Pa_{O_2} less than 60 mm Hg.
   b. *Physiologic shunt measurement.* An intrapulmonary shunt (Qsp/Qt) of less than 30% is desirable. A Qsp/Qt of between 10% to 20% is preferable.
   c. *Arterial oxyhemoglobin saturation.* Pulse oximeter (Sp_{O_2}) values of over 92% reflect adequate arterial oxygenation.
   d. *Physiologic deadspace measurement.* Because PPV increases deadspace ventilation, a V_D/V_T for patients on PPV of 50% to 60% is acceptable.
      Values of these indices of cardiopulmonary function that fall outside the desired ranges usually reflect a significant degree of pulmonary parenchymal disease. Discontinuing ventilatory support is seldom successful in the face of significant acute pulmonary parenchymal dysfunction.
3. Cardiovascular Assessment. Adequate cardiovascular function is required to sustain the spontaneous WOB. The following values are associated with adequate cardiovascular function.
   a. Heart rate of 60 to 100 beats/per minute with stable rhythm.
   b. Electrocardiogram showing no clinically significant arrhythmias.
   c. Stable blood pressure (BP) or mean arterial

pressure (MAP), which is not in the hypotensive range.

Assessment of Factors That May Increase Ventilatory Demand

Ventilatory demand is increased by elevated production of carbon dioxide ($\dot{V}co_2$), acidosis, hypoxemia and, to a lesser extent, by anemia. The following values are desirable.

1. Hemoglobin concentration of over 8 g/dL.
2. Nutritional support. Hyperalimentation increases $\dot{V}co_2$. Evaluate total calorie supply and mix of calorie substrates. Overfeeding (excessive calories) and feeding predominant carbohydrate calorie sources are undesirable and are often associated with $\dot{V}co_2$ of over 300 mL/min. Most critically ill patients do not require more than 35 kcal/kg ideal body weight. A mixed calorie source of 50:50 carbohydrate-to-fat is associated with the lowest respiratory quotient ($RQ = \dot{V}co_2/\dot{V}o_2$) and hence minimal $\dot{V}co_2$. See Chapter 16 for further discussion of the calorie needs of the critically ill patient).
3. Fever. An elevated metabolic rate will increase ventilatory demand.

Equipment

1. Manual ventilator with appropriate oxygen source and F_{IO_2}.
2. Spirometer.
3. Negative inspiratory force meter.

Required Monitoring

1. Electrocardiogram.
2. Blood pressure via arterial line or BP cuff.
3. Pulse oximeter.
4. Capnograph (optional).
5. Transcutaneous carbon dioxide monitor (optional).

Required Laboratory Data

1. Hemoglobin concentration.
2. Arterial blood gas analysis.

PROCEDURE

1. Introduce yourself to the patient.
2. Psychological preparation of the patient
   a. Fully explain ventilator discontinuance procedure to patient.
   b. Explain that discontinuing the ventilator is tailored to patient tolerance and that in some patients ventilator discontinuance is easily and quickly achieved, whereas others may need a longer weaning process. Therefore, the patient should not be discouraged if the first attempt is not successful.
   c. Reassure the patient that you will maintain close surveillance during the process and that he/she need not be fearful.
3. Ensure that all respiratory depressant and neuromuscular blocking medications have been reversed.
4. Select the technique to be used: ventilatory challenge or gradual weaning.
5. Ventilatory challenge. The initial transition from mechanical to spontaneous ventilation is accomplished best with a manual ventilator delivering 50% to 80% oxygen. This procedure directly and immediately involves you in the process and reassures the patient that you can breathe for him or her at any time if necessary.
   a. Disconnect the patient from the ventilator and augment the patient's spontaneous ventilation with a manual resuscitator.
   b. Provide a positive-pressure breath synchronized with the patient's spontaneous pattern of breathing approximately every 30 seconds. This procedure allows for a gradual, predictable, and

safe increase in $Paco_2$ and provides reassurance for the patient while he or she assumes the WOB.

  c. Monitor the patient's vital signs and clinical status.

    (1) Anticipate an increase in RR, V_T, BP/MAP, pulse rate, and possibly onset of slight diaphoresis as patient assumes the WOB.

    (2) Attempt to differentiate between physiologic and psychologic stress.

    (3) Remain at the patient's bedside for the first 15 minutes.

  d. If more than one breath every 30 seconds is required or the patient manifests significant detrimental changes in vital signs or clinical appearance, **reinstitute mechanical ventilation.**

  e. If the patient maintains stable cardiopulmonary function after 10 to 15 minutes, attach an appropriate circuit with fresh gas source to the endotracheal tube and observe.

  f. Measure arterial blood gases after 15 minutes to verify the adequacy of ventilation and arterial oxygenation.

6. Gradual weaning.

  a. Establish baseline values of vital signs, any hemodynamic measures available, and ABG analysis.

  b. Select ventilator mode: intermittent mandatory ventilation/synchronized IMV (IMV/SIMV), or pressure support (PS) ventilation.

    (1) The IMV/SIMV mode.

      (a) Decrease ventilator rate by two breaths per minute and observe the patient for 2 to 4 hours.

      (b) If cardiopulmonary function remains stable and ABG values are acceptable, reduce ventilator rate by a further two breaths per minute.

      (c) Continue this process until the patient is either weaned on to CPAP or manifests unstable cardiopulmonary function. If the patient manifests unstable cardiopulmonary function, increase the ventilator rate to a level associated with stable cardiopulmonary function and re-evaluate the indication for discontinuing ventilatory support.

   (2) The PS mode.

      (a) Stabilize the patient on PS ventilation (see Chapter 22).

      (b) Decrease the level of PS by 3 to 5 cm H_2O and observe the patient for 2 to 4 hours.

      (c) If cardiopulmonary function remains stable and ABG are acceptable, continue decremental reduction in PS level until the patient is either weaned onto a pressure support of 3 to 5 cm H_2O with or without CPAP or manifests unstable cardiopulmonary function. If unstable cardiopulmonary function develops, either increase the pressure support to a level associated with stable function or return the patient to conventional PPV and re-evaluate.

7. During ventilator discontinuance, maintaining support of pulmonary oxygen transfer is important. During the process of ventilator discontinuance, ensure that the FIO_2 is at least the same as the maintenance FIO_2 on the ventilator. If the PEEP/CPAP on the ventilator is greater than 5 cm H_2O, the manual ventilator should be adapted to provide the same level of PEEP/CPAP.

8. After discontinuing PPV, provide appropriate FIO_2, CPAP, and possibly PS by means of the endotracheal tube. In the intubated, spontaneously ventilating patient, 3 to 5 cm H_2O CPAP and 3 to 5 cm H_2O of PS help to maintain the functional residual capacity and minimize airway resistance secondary to the endotracheal tube.

FOLLOW-UP

1. Evaluate the stability of cardiopulmonary function of the spontaneously breathing patient after ventilator discontinuance for the first few hours. The frequency of these evaluations will depend on the clinical circumstances of each patient. Patients who maintain stable cardiopulmonary function while breathing spontaneously for 4 to 8 hours after discontinuance of PPV seldom require reinstitution of PPV.
2. Extubation of the patient is a clinical issue that is not necessarily tied to discontinuance of ventilatory support. Once a patient is breathing spontaneously, the need for an airway should be evaluated. Patients require artificial airways for one of the following reasons.
   a. Maintenance of airway.
   b. Protection of airway.
   c. Provision of airway pressure therapy.
   d. Facilitation of bronchial hygiene.
3. If no indication for intubation is present, extubate the patient and provide appropriate F_{IO_2} by face mask or nasal cannula.

COMPLICATIONS

Failure of the patient to maintain adequate cardiopulmonary function while breathing spontaneously must be carefully evaluated.

1. Check for iatrogenic reasons for the failure, such as oversedation, inadequate reversal of neuromuscular blocking drugs, failure to provide appropriate support of oxygenation, use of a breathing circuit with high intrinsic airway resistance, or equipment malfunction.
2. Check for reversible factors that may be increasing the ventilatory demand, such as acidemia, hypox-

emia, anemia, provision of excess calories, or inappro-
priate calorie source.

When these factors have been ruled out and clinical
assessment of cardiopulmonary reserves still indicates
that the patient should be able to breathe spontaneously, the assumption must be made that the patient is
either unable to come off the ventilator because the underlying disease that led to a need for ventilatory support is not reversed adequately, or that psychologic dependence exists. Most weaning problems are due to

1. Attempting to discontinue ventilation too early in
the disease course.
2. Improper ventilator maintenance.
3. Pre-existing chronic disease or malnutrition that
severely limits cardiopulmonary reserves.

In the absence of these, the next most common problem
is psychologic dependence.

A few patients may require reinstitution of partial
ventilatory support at night because they are afraid to
fall asleep breathing on their own. This approach may
be a reasonable approach for several days. Psychologic
dependence is a difficult problem and one that demands a great deal of understanding and patience.
These individuals are in need of a weaning process in
the traditional sense, that is, the process of taking the
patient off the ventilator for short periods of time and
trying progressively to lengthen the periods off PPV.

DOCUMENTATION

Write a note in the patient's chart that includes

1. Baseline values of cardiopulmonary function.
2. Justification for your judgment that the primary
pathology is adequately reversed.

3. Justification for choice of technique for discontinuance of PPV.

4. Description of what was actually done and outcome.

5. Clinical decision regarding extubation.

In addition write orders for

1. Type of breathing circuit patient was placed on after successful discontinuance of PPV.

2. Fraction of inspired oxygen.

3. CPAP and PS level (if any).

4. Frequency of ABG monitoring and "Call Physician" parameters for the ABG results.

SUGGESTED READING

MacIntyre NR: Weaning from mechanical ventilatory support: volume assisting intermittent breaths versus pressure assisting every breath, *Respir Care* 33:121, 1988.

Shapiro BA, Cane RD: Conventional mechanical ventilation. In Cane RD, Shapiro BA, Davison R, editors: *Case studies in critical care medicine,* ed 2, St Louis, 1990, Mosby–Year Book, pp 52–81.

24

PEEP/CPAP
Therapy

Jukka Räsänen, M.D.

INTRODUCTION

Regardless of cause, acute parenchymal lung injury frequently results in a reduction in the gas volume of the lung. The loss in lung volume effects

1. A decrease in the distensibility of the lung parenchyma
2. A narrowing of the airways
3. A reduction in the caliber of large pulmonary blood vessels.

The clinical pulmonary manifestations of these pathophysiological changes include

1. Impairment in arterial blood oxygenation
2. Increased work of breathing
3. In extreme cases, accumulation of carbon dioxide with respiratory acidemia.

Other organ systems, such as the heart, are affected secondarily but nevertheless significantly. Positive airway pressure therapy is used in an attempt to reinflate the lung close to its original volume in order to minimize detrimental effects. The term positive end-expiratory pressure (PEEP) is usually used to denote positive end-expiratory airway pressure in conjunction with positive pressure mechanical ventilation. The term continuous positive airway pressure (CPAP) denotes use of positive airway pressure during spontaneous breathing to elevate airway pressure to a prescribed level for the entire duration of the ventilatory cycle. This terminology has been adopted because the use of PEEP in a spontaneously breathing patient, although possible, may be hazardous and is never used intentionally in patients with acute respiratory failure (Fig 24–1).

OBJECTIVE

The primary objectives of PEEP/CPAP therapy are

1. To increase arterial blood oxygenation and tissue oxygen delivery by improving the ventilation/perfusion relationships in the lung.

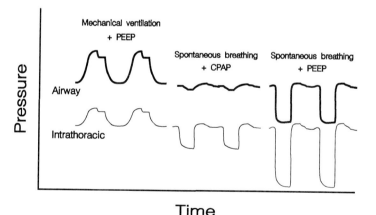

FIG 24–1.
Changes in airway *(thick line)* and intrathoracic *(thin line)* pressures during mechanical ventilation with PEEP and during spontaneous breathing with PEEP and CPAP. The fall in airway pressure during spontaneous breathing with PEEP requires the patient to effect an equivalent decrease in intrathoracic pressure, which increases ventilatory work.

2. To decrease the work of breathing by increasing lung compliance and decreasing airway resistance.

Secondary objectives, dependent upon attainment of the primary objectives, include reduction in inspired oxygen concentration (FIO_2) and the level of mechanical ventilatory support.

Indications

The use of PEEP/CPAP therapy is indicated

1. To correct hypoxemia secondary to existence of areas with low ventilation/perfusion ratio or true intra-pulmonary shunting in the lungs.
2. To improve lung compliance secondary to loss of intrathoracic gas volume.

Contraindications

1. Severe hypovolemia.
2. Hemodynamically significant pericardial tampon-ade.
3. Untreated tension pneumothorax.
4. Application of CPAP with a mask is contraindi-cated in the absence of protective airway reflexes.

PREPARATION

Equipment

All modern ventilators have an adjustment enabling administration of PEEP during controlled mechanical ventilation. If a ventilator is not available, PEEP can be administered by attaching a PEEP valve to the exhala-tion port of a self-inflating resuscitator bag.

The demands for the characteristics of the breathing circuit are much greater during administration of CPAP, that is, when CPAP is to be applied while the pa-tient is breathing spontaneously. Two basic circuit con-figurations are used for administering CPAP.

1. In a continuous-flow CPAP system, a high flow of gas is delivered into the circuit and allowed to exit through a threshold resistor valve. The opening pressure of the valve determines the pressure in the circuit and in the patient's airway. If the continuous flow rate matches or exceeds the patient's peak inspiratory flow, the airway pressure will remain constant throughout the spontaneous respiratory cycle. The circuit flow can be decreased if a reservoir bag is added to the inspiratory limb of the breathing circuit to provide an additional source of gas during the inspiratory phase. However, the size and the compliance characteristics of this bag have to be such that partial deflation of the bag during inspiration does not result in an appreciable decrease in the circuit pressure.

2. In a demand-flow CPAP circuit, gas is supplied to the patient only during inspiration. To initiate gas flow in the beginning of the inspiratory phase, the patient is required to generate a decrease in airway pressure. This transient airway pressure drop will be sensed by the breathing circuit, which will respond by opening the inspiratory demand valve to initiate gas flow. To avoid unnecessary respiratory effort related to changes in airway pressure, the circuit pressure should remain within ± 2 cm H_2O of the prescribed level during spontaneous breathing with CPAP. This goal is frequently not achieved with demand-flow circuits because of the insensitivity of the demand valve and the time lag between the triggering effort and the opening of the valve. An insensitive demand valve requires a large fall in airway and intrathoracic pressure before flow is initiated, reflected by an early inspiratory drop in airway pressure with signs of increased early inspiratory effort on examination of the patient.

An inspiratory fall in airway and intrathoracic pressure during breathing with continuous-flow CPAP circuits frequently results from inadequate inspiratory flow. However, the characteristics of the expiratory valve are also important in assuring minimum work of breathing. Characteristics of expiratory valves range from a flow resistor in which the pressure gradient across the valve varies with flow through the valve, to threshold resistors in which the pressure gradient is stable within a wide range of flows. Use of flow-resistor expiratory valves result in fluctuation in circuit pressure when flow through the valve varies during the different phases of the respiratory cycle. This variation will result in an inspiratory drop and an expiratory overshoot of airway pressure with respect to the prescribed level of CPAP (Fig 24–2).

Those who prescribe PEEP or CPAP therapy must know the capabilities and limitations of the available equipment. Frequently, apparent intolerance of the work of spontaneous breathing results from unfavorable mechanical characteristics of the breathing circuit and not from factors intrinsic to the patient's respiratory system. In these cases, removal of unnecessary deadspace and resistance-producing parts such as acute angles and in-line foam humidifiers and, if necessary, switching to a continuous-flow

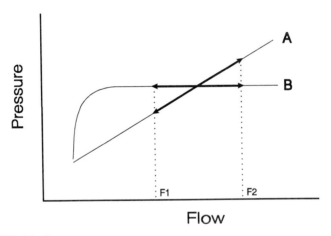

FIG 24–2.
Changes in circuit pressure during alteration in flow through a flow resistor *(A)* and a threshold resistor *(B)* exhalation valve. Fluctuations in circuit flow between *F1* and *F2* during the ventilatory cycle effect a concomitant fluctuation in circuit pressure if the exhalation valve is a flow resistor. If a threshold resistor is used, circuit pressure remains stable.

breathing circuit may make the difference between success and failure.

Required Monitoring

Monitoring during PEEP/CPAP therapy is necessary to document favorable effects on pulmonary gas exchange and lung mechanics and to detect possible impairment in cardiovascular performance or other organ function.

1. *Arterial oxygenation.* Blood gas analysis or pulse oximetry can be used to detect changes in arterial blood oxygenation.

2. *Lung mechanics.* The effects of PEEP/CPAP on lung mechanics can be assessed only by observing the clinical indicators of ventilatory work such as the patient's breathing pattern, respiratory rate, use of ventilatory muscles, and suprasternal or intercostal retractions.

3. *Ventilation.* The effects of elevated airway pressure on ventilatory function may be assessed with end-tidal, transcutaneous, or arterial carbon dioxide tension measurements.

4. *Work of breathing.* The patient's heart rate and blood pressure should be monitored to detect and document relief of cardiovascular stress secondary to decreasing the work of breathing, or to detect impairment in cardiovascular performance secondary to increased intrathoracic pressure.

5. *Cardiovascular function.* In patients with known or expected cardiovascular instability, monitoring of filling pressures, cardiac output, and mixed venous oxyhemoglobin saturation with a pulmonary artery catheter is recommended strongly. Patients receiving PEEP/CPAP levels higher than 15 cm H_2O should probably be monitored routinely with a pulmonary artery catheter.

Required Laboratory Data

   A.B.G. analysis.

PROCEDURE

Application of CPAP With a Mask

1. Before application of mask-CPAP, perform a well-focused, brief clinical examination to evaluate the following.
   a. Ventilatory work.
   b. Arterial blood oxygenation.
   c. Adequacy of ventilation.
   d. Volume status.
   e. Level of consciousness.
   f. Oxygen therapy.
2. Briefly explain the procedure to the patient.
3. Assemble the breathing circuit and test for appropriate operation, F_{IO_2}, and circuit pressure. Occlusion of CPAP valves after cleaning is common; all CPAP valves should be tested for adequate opening pressure prior to use. The initial F_{IO_2} should be the same as that given to the patient before CPAP therapy, and the initial CPAP level should be one-half that assumed to be adequate for the patient, or 5 to 10 cm H_2O.
4. After initiation of full flow in the breathing circuit, manually place the mask to a gentle seal on the patient's face. Then comfort and encourage the patient to help him/her adapt to the breathing circuit.
5. Simultaneously, observe ventilatory mechanics and the pulse oximeter for evidence of improvement or impairment. Initial changes in oxygenation and lung mechanics usually are observed by both the physician and the patient within 2 to 3 minutes of mask placement. If response is favorable, as evidenced by improved oxygenation and/or decreased work of breathing, attach the mask in place with straps.

6. Thereafter, reduce the circuit flow to a minimum that will still prevent fluctuations in airway pressure greater than ±2 cm H_2O.

7. Titrate CPAP to its final level in small increments of 2 to 3 cm H_2O with close observation of oxygenation, ventilatory mechanics, and cardiovascular performance. The definition of optimum CPAP is controversial. Some authors favor application of the lowest level of CPAP that will produce adequate arterial blood oxygenation [(Sp_{O_2}) greater than 90%] when Fi_{O_2} is 0.50, whereas others advocate increase in airway pressure until the intrapulmonary shunt fraction no longer decreases. Still other authorities propose titration of CPAP to maximum oxygen delivery, maximum lung compliance, or minimum respiratory deadspace volume. If invasive monitoring is available, increase the CPAP level until oxygen delivery no longer improves in relation to oxygen consumption, or until no further improvement in respiratory mechanics can be observed. In the absence of invasive monitoring, the more conservative approach of ensuring adequate oxygenation with nontoxic Fi_{O_2} of less than 0.50 is recommended.

The effects of CPAP on gas exchange and lung mechanics do not always occur simultaneously and to the same degree. Therefore, one or the other may be emphasized in guiding CPAP therapy for a particular patient. The patient's subjective assessment should never be overlooked as a method of monitoring appropriate level of CPAP particularly when the objective of the treatment is to reduce the work of breathing.

An excessive level of CPAP can frequently be diagnosed from observation of the patient's respiratory mechanics at the bedside. The patient switches from a passive exhalation to an active exhalation in order to maintain a normal functional residual capacity, which the inappropriately high CPAP is trying to elevate. Depending on the patient's ventilatory reserve, the arterial carbon dioxide tension ($Paco_2$) may increase simultaneously. A level of CPAP that is excessive from a hemodynamic standpoint can be diagnosed only by measuring oxygen delivery. Arterial blood oxygenation may still be improving even though the elevated airway and intrathoracic pressures have reduced cardiac output and thereby impaired oxygen delivery.

PEEP/CPAP Therapy in Intubated Patients

Even in patients connected to ventilators, PEEP/CPAP therapy should not be used unless it is indicated to improve gas exchange or lung mechanics. Initiation of therapy and titration of the appropriate level of pressure follows the principles explained earlier in this chapter. Remember that many ventilator circuits have poor flow and resistance characteristics for spontaneous breathing. If the patient does not need mechanical ventilation, switching over to a stand-alone CPAP circuit frequently produces better results. If that is not possible, a low level of pressure support may be added to unsupported spontaneous breaths in order to overcome circuit resistance. Addition of PEEP to controlled mechanical ventilation will increase mean airway pressure by the amount of PEEP. However, the improvement in lung mechanics secondary to increase in lung volume produced by PEEP can often be used to reduce the amount of mechanical ventilatory support administered to the patient. Therefore, the net effect may be a decrease in intrathoracic pressure and potentially less cardiovascular compromise.

FOLLOW-UP

The use of PEEP/CPAP constitutes acute and temporary therapy that eventually will have to be discontinued. Furthermore, the patient's requirement of PEEP/CPAP changes over time periods that are sometimes measured in minutes. Therefore, the initial application of PEEP/CPAP must be followed by a plan to correct the underlying lung injury that brought about the requirement for respiratory support; to reassess the need and to readjust the level of PEEP/CPAP; and, ultimately, to wean and discontinue such therapy. Readjustment of PEEP/CPAP follows a monitoring approach similar to that used during initiation of therapy. In patients with both cardiovascular and pulmonary instability, repeated full cardiopulmonary assessment at different levels of airway pressure may be required at intervals determined by the clinical state of the patient. However, recent studies indicate that estimates of venous admixture and oxygen extraction ratio from continuous pulse and pulmonary artery oximetry, coupled with bedside clinical assessment of ventilatory mechanics, provide sufficiently accurate information for bedside titration of PEEP/CPAP.

Appropriate use of PEEP/CPAP allows a reduction in F_{IO_2} and mechanical ventilatory support in addition to correcting abnormalities in gas exchange and ventilatory mechanics. Support of lung volume with PEEP/CPAP often makes weaning the patient from oxygen therapy and mechanical ventilatory support easier. Weaning from PEEP/CPAP should occur after weaning from ventilatory support. It should proceed with the same vigilance used during initial application of elevated airway pressure. Because changes in intrathoracic pressure may induce significant shifts in intravascular volume, adjustment of cardiac and vasoactive medications, diuretics, and fluid infusion rates may be necessary to complement weaning from PEEP/CPAP.

COMPLICATIONS

1. *Increase in deadspace.* Hyperinflation of the alveoli by excessive airway pressure may prevent or inhibit blood flow so that large regions of the lung will be deadspace and will no longer participate in gas exchange. Depending on general ventilatory

reserves, this deadspace ventilation may effect an increase in Pa_{CO_2} and a widening of the end-tidal to arterial CO_2 tension (i.e. Pa-$_{ET}CO_2$) gradient.

2. *Increased ventilatory work.* In addition to an increased minute ventilatory requirement secondary to increased deadspace, overdistention of the rib cage will impair the patient's ability to breathe spontaneously as the resting thoracic volume increases toward the end-inspiratory level.

3. *Barotrauma.* Distention of the airways also may lead to structural damage, with resultant interstitial emphysema, pneumothorax, pneumomediastinum, pneumopericardium, pneumoperitoneum, and subcutaneous emphysema. Rupture of airways is more a function of excess volume than excess pressure. Therefore, barotrauma is seen more often when the pulmonary parenchymal disease is inhomogeneous, such as during the healing phase of acute lung injury. The role of airway pressure in producing such injury is still unclear. Since end-inspiratory lung volumes and pressures are much greater than the end-expiratory ones, positive pressure mechanical ventilation is more likely to cause barotrauma than PEEP/CPAP therapy.

4. *Cardiovascular instability.* The type and extent of cardiovascular complications of PEEP/CPAP therapy depend on the patient's initial cardiac and pulmonary function. The PEEP/CPAP therapy can produce changes in both preload and afterload.

   a. Right ventricular preload. Transmission of elevated airway pressure into the intrathoracic space and direct compression of the right side of the heart by the expanding lungs impede the return of venous blood to the right atrium. The reduction in venous return is reflected on the left side of the heart and will decrease left ventricular filling volume, stroke volume, and cardiac output in a normal preload-dependent circulatory system. This effect will be enhanced if the patient is hypovolemic.

b. Left ventricular afterload. The elevation of intrathoracic pressure subsequent to application of PEEP/CPAP will decrease left ventricular afterload as the pressure surrounding the heart increases. The beneficial effect of this afterload reduction is negligible in patients with normal cardiovascular function, but it may be significant in patients with failure of the left side of the heart. Therefore, the cardiovascular effects of PEEP/CPAP form a spectrum. The hypovolemic patient with normal left ventricular function will probably suffer a reduction in stroke volume and cardiac output with the application of PEEP/CPAP. However, the fluid-overloaded patient with severe congestive heart failure may benefit from the application of elevated airway pressure.

c. Right ventricular afterload. Because lung volume is a major determinant of pulmonary vascular resistance, the application of PEEP/CPAP has an effect of right ventricular afterload. If PEEP/CPAP is used appropriately to correct reduced gas volume of the lung, pulmonary vascular resistance will be minimized. However, if the lungs are hyperinflated, increased pulmonary vascular resistance and afterloading of the right ventricle will result.

Monitoring of cardiovascular function is also confounded by the application of PEEP/CPAP therapy. Vascular pressure measurements made from inside the thoracic cavity are traditionally referenced to atmospheric pressure. When the pressure surrounding these structures is raised by the application of positive airway pressure, the pressures so derived no longer accurately represent the transmural filling pressures of these structures. To account for the effect of PEEP/CPAP on intrathoracic vascular pressure measurements, for most clinical situations subtract 50% of the end-expiratory airway pressure from the intrathoracic vascular pressure values referenced to atmospheric pressure and measured at end-expiration.

5. *Other organ dysfunction.* Complications of PEEP/CPAP therapy seen in other organ systems usually reflect in hemodynamics.

   a. Renal effects. Impairment in renal function seen with PEEP/CPAP is believed to be secondary to decreased renal blood flow, increased renal venous pressure, and intrarenal redistribution of blood flow.

   b. Gastrointestinal effects. Impairment in the regional perfusion of intra-abdominal organs by increased intrathoracic pressure has been suspected, but is not well documented.

   c. Central nervous system effects. Impairment of cerebral blood flow during PEEP/CPAP therapy may occur because of reduction in mean arterial pressure and elevation in jugular venous pressure. However, the effects of PEEP on intracranial pressure are inconsistent and do not warrant exclusion of PEEP/CPAP from the treatment of patients with elevated intracranial pressure, if such therapy is indicated to improve pulmonary function. In these cases, it is advisable to use intracranial pressure monitoring to detect possible detrimental effects of elevated airway pressure on cerebral perfusion pressure.

6. *Mask-related complications.* Apart from complications of elevated airway pressure itself, the application of CPAP with a mask has its own potential complications.

   a. The most common complication is skin breakdown under the areas of mask contact. To minimize the incidence of pressure sores, avoid tight binding of the mask and increase the breathing circuit flow to compensate for gas leak from under the mask, which occurs commonly.

   b. Drying of the oropharyngeal airway may occur if appropriate humidification of the inspired gas is not arranged.

   c. Aspiration of gastric contents is an immediate

serious threat if mask-CPAP therapy is used in a patient without protective airway reflexes. However, in awake patients, use of mask-CPAP does not in itself induce nausea or vomiting, and application of this therapy does not routinely require placement of a nasogastric tube.

d. Inadvertent loss of CPAP upon mask displacement or disconnection may suddenly effect a deterioration in the patients arterial blood oxygenation and an increase in the work of breathing. Therefore, patients receiving PEEP/CPAP therapy, even during spontaneous breathing without an artificial airway, should be closely monitored in an intensive care unit.

DOCUMENTATION

All decisions regarding initiation, discontinuation, and adjustment of PEEP/CPAP and the rationale behind these decisions should be clearly indicated in the patient's medical records. Because the application of positive airway pressure affects most organ systems, other medical specialists may be involved in the care of the patient. Therefore, communication between physicians and coordination and synchronization of therapy are essential. The order for PEEP/CPAP therapy should define the equipment to be used and the pressure level. When CPAP is administered intermittently with a mask, the order should indicate the prescribed duration and frequency of its application.

SUGGESTED READING

Miro AM et al: Hemodynamic effects of mechanical ventilation. In Grenvik A et al, editors: *Contemporary management in critical care*, New York, 1991, Churchill Livingstone, pp 73–90.

Shapiro BA et al: CPAP/PEEP therapy. In *Clinical application of respiratory care*, ed 4, St Louis, 1991, Mosby–Year Book, pp 335–364.

25

Transvenous Cardiac Pacing

Jeffrey Goldberger, M.D.
Alan Kadish, M.D.

INTRODUCTION

Temporary pacing of the heart has developed over the last 30 to 40 years as an important therapeutic modality in patients with bradyarrhythmias and as a prophylactic treatment for patients at risk for progression to serious bradyarrhythmias and heart block. Three primary modalities are available for temporary cardiac pacing:

1. Placement of a transvenous pacing catheter.
2. A transthoracic catheter (see chapter 26).
3. The use of external electrodes on the skin for pacing (see chapter 27).

Each modality has advantages and disadvantages. When the need for cardiac pacing arises, the physician caring for the patient must carefully weigh the risks and benefits of each of these pacing modalities.

OBJECTIVE

Successfully pace the heart with a transvenous pacing catheter.

Indications

1. Bradyarrhythmias associated with acute myocardial infarction.
   a. Symptomatic bradycardia or heart block.
   b. Second-degree atrioventricular (AV) block, Mobitz type 2.
   c. Other high-grade AV block.
   d. Complete heart block—except in asymptomatic patient with acute inferior wall myocardial infarction.
   e. New bifascicular block.
   f. Pre-existing bifascicular block with new PR interval prolongation.
   g. Alternating bundle branch block.
2. Bradyarrhythmias not associated with acute myocardial infarction.
   a. Symptomatic bradyarrhythmias and/or heart block.
   b. Complete heart block with a wide QRS escape rhythm.
   c. Asystole.
3. Tachyarrhythmias
   a. Antitachycardia pacing in patients with recurrent ventricular or supraventricular tachycardia while other therapeutic options are being implemented.
   b. Prevention of bradycardia or pauses in patients with bradycardia-dependent ventricular arrhythmias, such as drug-induced torsades de pointes.

Contraindications

1. Bradycardia associated with hypothermia.

PREPARATION

Emergency temporary cardiac pacing can be achieved with either ventricular, sequential AV, or on rare occasions, atrial pacing. Ventricular pacing is the technique of choice in most circumstances. However, sequential AV pacing is required when maintenance of an adequate cardiac output is dependent on atrial systole, such as a patient with a hemodynamically significant right ventricular infarction. Each is discussed separately, giving preparation and procedure.

A. VENTRICULAR PACING

Equipment

1. Materials to obtain central venous access (see Chapter 2).
2. Either a 5 or 6 F stiff bipolar pacing catheter, or a 4 or 5 F flexible balloon-flotation bipolar pacing catheter.
3. Cables to connect the pacing catheter to the pulse generator and to the V lead of an electrocardiogram machine (alligator clips work well).
4. Fluoroscopy is desirable, though not essential.
5. An electrocardiogram (EKG) recorder.
6. A pulse generator (with a new battery) that is the pacing unit (Fig 25–1).
7. Defibrillator.

Required Monitoring

None.

Required Laboratory Data

1. If time permits, a prothrombin time, partial thromboplastin time, and platelet count should be ob-

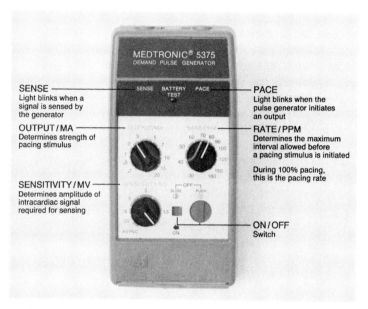

FIG 25–1.
Pulse generator for temporary transvenous pacing.

tained to help determine the most appropriate route
and site for central venous access (see Chapter 2).

2. Serum electrolytes.

3. Arterial blood gases or pulse oximetry.

VENTRICULAR PACING PROCEDURE

1. Before implementing transvenous cardiac pacing,
   correct any pre-existing arterial hypoxemia or
   serum electrolyte abnormalities.

2. To secure central venous access, place an
   introducer sheath into the central venous system
   (see Chapter 2). The right internal jugular vein and
   left subclavian vein allow the pacing catheter to
   be manipulated into the right ventricle with
   greatest ease. The femoral vein or median cubital

vein (preferably left) can also be used for placement of a transvenous pacing catheter. The right subclavian vein is the least desirable site because of the acute angle at which it joins the brachiocephalic vein. The choice of access site will depend on the clinical situation. If the patient is at extremely high risk of bleeding, the median cubital vein, accessed either percutaneously or by surgical cut-down, is preferred.

3. Wash your hands and don mask, sterile gown, and gloves. Observe strict aseptic technique during venous access and passage of the pacing catheter. Good aseptic technique increases the time the catheter can remain safely in place and decreases the incidence of infection.

4. Once an introducer sheath has been placed in the central venous system, fluoroscopic or EKG guidance can be used to position the pacing catheter.

   a. *Fluoroscopic guidance*
      (1) Advance the pacing catheter through the venous sheath with fluoroscopic guidance.
         (a) With flexible, balloon-flotation catheters, inflate the balloon once the catheter is in the central venous system. Blood flow will direct the catheter into the right ventricle. When the catheter crosses the tricuspid valve into the right ventricle, deflate the balloon and position the catheter in the right ventricular apex.
         (b) When employing a stiff catheter, use fluoroscopic guidance to advance the catheter into the right atrium and then position it to advance into the right ventricle. The catheter may need to be torqued so that it points in the correct direction to cross the tricuspid valve. The right ventricle lies anterior to the right atrium. Therefore, if the catheter is pointing toward the lateral right atrial

wall, it will require counterclockwise torque (if the wire is passed by way of the superior vena cava). When the catheter crosses the tricuspid valve, advance it to the right ventricular apex.

(2) Once the catheter is positioned at the apex of the right ventricle, check the adequacy of the site for cardiac pacing (discussed later).

b. *Electrocardiographic guidance.* If fluoroscopy is not available, only a balloon-flotation catheter should be used. Blind passage of a stiff catheter might result in intravascular or intracardiac injury.

(1) Connect the limb leads of an electrocardiogram machine to the patient in the standard fashion.

(2) Attach the distal tip of the pacing catheter (labeled either distal or negative) with alligator clips to the V lead of the electrocardiogram machine. Turn on the EKG machine and set it to record the V lead, which will reflect intracavitary potentials via the pacing catheter. Ideally, record a surface EKG lead simultaneously with the intracardiac recording so that intracardiac atrial and ventricular electrograms can be easily identified by correlation with the P wave and QRS complex respectively.

(3) Advance the pacing catheter through the venous introducer sheath until it is in the central venous system.

(4) Inflate the balloon. The V lead recording will resemble the tracing shown in Figure 25–2,A.

(5) Advance the catheter into the right atrium. The V lead recordings will appear as in Figure 25–2,B. Note the sharp, prominent atrial deflections, in addition to a relatively small ventricular component.

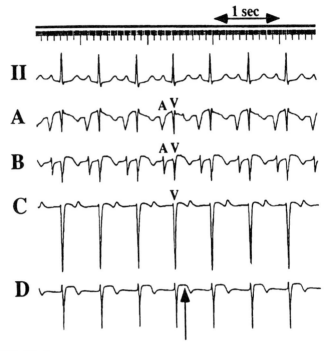

FIG 25–2.
Simultaneous recordings of surface electrocardiographic *lead II* with intracardiac unipolar recordings from the junction of the superior vena cava
and right atrium *(A)*, the mid-right atrium *(B)*, the ventricular cavity *(C)*, and
a ventricular endocardial recording *(D)*. No atrial deflection is noted on the
recordings made in the right ventricle. Note the ST segment elevation in
the endocardial ventricular recording *(arrow)*. A = atrial depolarization;
V = ventricular depolarization.

    (6) Advance the catheter into the right
        ventricle. Once the pacing catheter has
        entered the right atrium, it should cross the
        tricuspid annulus after being advanced an
        additional 5 to 10 cm. As the catheter
        crosses the tricuspid valve, the V lead
        tracing will show a large intracavitary
        ventricular depolarization, with minimal or
        no atrial deflections (Fig 25–2,C).
    (7) When the catheter is in the ventricle, deflate
        the balloon and advance the catheter until

it contacts the right ventricular myocardium. Myocardial contact is confirmed by the development of an injury potential or what appears to be ST segment elevation in the V lead tracing (Fig 25–2,D).
5. Confirm pacing catheter position. Ideally, the pacing catheter should be positioned in the right ventricular apex, as this is the most stable site and the catheter will dislodge less frequently than from any other site. Aside from the right ventricle, the pacing catheter may come to lie in one of four possible positions.

a. *Coronary sinus.* If the catheter is advanced into the coronary sinus, the V lead recordings will generally show a sharp atrial potential and a ventricular depolarization as shown in Figure 25–3,A. When the catheter is in the coronary sinus, it is possible to advance it into one of the posterior descending veins. It might feel as though the catheter is up against a wall and ventricular depolarizations may be recorded. Furthermore, ventricular pacing may be possible. However, an injury current will not be identified. A good clue that the catheter has been advanced into the coronary sinus can be obtained by examining the relationship of the atrial electrogram to the P wave. Since the coronary sinus lies in the AV groove between the left atrium and left ventricle, a catheter in the coronary sinus records left atrial activity and the atrial electrogram tracing will be noted during the late portion (toward the end) of the P wave (Fig 25–3,A). In contrast, the atrial electrogram from a catheter in the right atrium will occur during the early portion of the P wave.

b. *Inferior vena cava.* The catheter can be advanced into the inferior vena cava. In this case, the electrograms will change from large intra-atrial cavitary potentials to a recording of

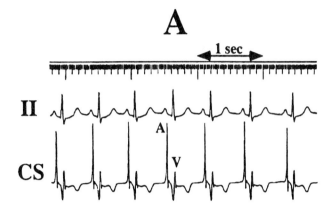

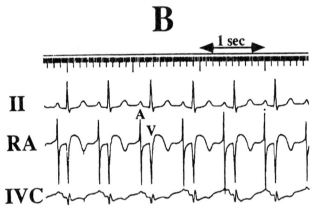

FIG 25–3.
Simultaneous recordings of surface electrocardiographic *lead II* with intra-cardiac unipolar recordings made from the coronary sinus *(panel A)* and recordings made from the right atrium and inferior vena cava *(panel B)*. Note the marked diminution in electrogram amplitude when the catheter exits the heart into the inferior vena cava. In the recordings made from the coronary sinus the atrial electrogram occurs toward the end of the P wave, whereas in the recordings made from the right atrium, the atrial electro-gram occurs towards the beginning of the P wave. *A* = atrial depolariza-tion; *V* = ventricular depolarization.

a low-amplitude P wave and QRS complexes as shown in Figure 25–3,B.

c. *Right atrium.* The catheter may coil in the right atrium, in which case persistent right atrial electrograms will be obtained.

d. *Left atrium or ventricle.* The catheter may cross an atrial septal defect or a patent foramen ovale into the left atrium and then into the left ventricle. The EKG characteristics will appear as in Figure 25–2, with the paced QRS morphology showing a right bundle branch block pattern on the 12-lead EKG. To confirm catheter placement in the left heart, obtain anteroposterior (AP) and lateral chest roentgenograms.

In any of these situations, withdraw the catheter and re-advance to position it in the right ventricle. If repeated attempts at right ventricular catheter placement are unsuccessful (such as may occur in patients with significant tricuspid regurgitation or severely depressed cardiac output), fluoroscopic guidance is recommended. Use of a stiffer pacing catheter may facilitate proper placement.

6. Confirm adequate pacing function. Once you have placed the catheter with either technique, check the pacemaker function to confirm proper positioning. The pacemaker pulse generator has two functions: monitoring cardiac rhythm to determine the need for pacing (sensing), and initiating an output (pacing). Therefore, the two pacing parameters to check and set are the pacing threshold and the sensing threshold.

a. *Pacing threshold.* The pacing threshold is the minimum current (in milliamperes) required to successfully capture (or pace) the right ventricle. To determine the pacing threshold, select the asynchronous pacing mode and set the pulse generator to a rate significantly faster (usually 10 to 20 beats depending on the clinical situation) than the patient's intrinsic heart rate (see Figure 25–1). Set the pacemaker output to the minimum value and turn on the pulse generator. Slowly increase the output until ventricular capture is obtained. The pacing threshold is the minimum current that results in ventricular capture.

The pacing threshold should be less than 1 mamp. If it is significantly higher, there is either poor contact of the pacing catheter with the endocardium or the site is not suitable for pacing. If the pacing threshold is greater than 1 mamp, slightly advance the pacing catheter. If the pacing threshold does not significantly improve, reposition the catheter to another site. To provide an adequate safety margin, set the pacing output at 2 to 3 times the threshold. Observe the heart rhythm closely during threshold testing as ventricular arrhythmias, particularly ventricular fibrillation in patients with significant bradycardia, can occur. If emergency pacing is required, it will be impossible to check the pacing threshold. As soon as the pacing catheter is in position, initiate pacing. Once the patient's condition has stabilized, check the pacing threshold.

b. *Sensing threshold.* The sensitivity dial on the pulse generator (see Fig 25–1) helps determine the amplitude of the ventricular electrogram that the pulse generator will consider to be a ventricular event (or beat). The pulse generator measures the amplitude of the ventricular electrogram recorded from the distal and proximal electrodes of the pacing catheter, which does not necessarily correlate with the surface QRS amplitude. When the sensitivity dial is turned toward the higher numbers, the pulse generator is less sensitive to the patient's own intrinsic ventricular depolarizations. At an amplitude greater than 20 mV, the device is virtually functioning in an asynchronous mode: that is, it cannot sense the patient's intrinsic ventricular depolarizations. When the sensitivity is turned to the minimum value, the pulse generator is maximally sensitive to the patient's intrinsic ventricular activity. Although, with the sensitivity set at minimum, the pulse generator will almost certainly sense the patient's intrinsic ventricular depolarizations, it may also sense other electrical signals such as T waves, muscle activity, and electrical noise.

If the patient has an adequate intrinsic rhythm, determine the sensing threshold. Set the pacing rate below the patient's intrinsic rate and the sensitivity to the minimum value. There is a small light at the top of the pulse generator that blinks whenever a QRS complex is sensed by the device [it is labeled "SENSE" (see Figure 25–1)]. Observe the sensing light and slowly increase the sensitivity; the pulse generator will eventually stop sensing the patient's intrinsic ventricular depolarization. The maximum number on the sensitivity dial at which the QRS is still sensed is the sensing threshold.

The appropriate sensitivity level setting depends on the clinical situation. The pulse generator can be set to pace continuously, termed asynchronous pacing, or to pace only when the patient's intrinsic ventricular rate falls below a preselected rate, termed demand pacing. For demand pacing, set the sensitivity to one half of the threshold level and adjust if either oversensing (that is, T waves inhibit pacemaker output) or undersensing occurs [that is, the pacer fails to sense a premature ventricular contraction (PVC) that might have a smaller amplitude than the normal ventricular contraction]. Remember, the amplitude of the surface recording of either a PVC or a normally conducted beat is not necessarily related to the intracardiac ventricular electrogram detected by the pulse generator.

7. Following measurement of sensing and pacing thresholds, obtain a 12-lead EKG during ventricular pacing. Pacing in the right ventricular apex produces a left bundle branch block morphology with a *superior axis.* Pacing of sites other than the right ventricle will probably show a left bundle branch block morphology with a *different axis* because the right ventricle is activated before the left. If the paced QRS complex has a right bundle branch morphology, pacing from either the left ventricle or one of the posterior descending veins should be suspected. Rarely, a right bundle branch morphology may be observed as a normal finding of pacing the right ventricle.

8. If the patient has a stable underlying cardiac rhythm, record a bipolar and unipolar tracing from the pacing electrodes. Slowly decrease the pacing rate until the patient's intrinsic rhythm returns. When the patient is no longer paced, turn off the pulse generator.

   a. *Unipolar electrogram.* Connect the negative or distal electrode of the pacing catheter to the V lead of the EKG machine and record the unipolar electrogram.

   b. *Bipolar electrogram.* Connect the negative or distal electrode of the pacing catheter to the left arm connection of the EKG machine and connect the positive or proximal electrode of the pacing catheter to the right arm connection of the EKG machine. Record lead I, which will show the bipolar electrogram that the pulse generator (pacemaker) is actually seeing. To measure the amplitude of the bipolar electrogram, apply a calibration marker from the EKG machine. The peak-to-peak amplitude of the bipolar electrogram should correlate with the measured sensitivity threshold. The unipolar and bipolar electrograms are useful for evaluation of changes during follow-up (discussed later).

Obtain all the discussed measurements only in patients with *stable cardiac rhythms* during placement of a temporary pacing catheter. Clearly, there are situations in which it is not feasible to obtain all these measurements and recordings. Use clinical judgement when determining which measurements to obtain.

9. Once all of the appropriate measurements have been obtained, securely fix the pacing catheter to the skin with a stitch and/or steristrips. Apply a sterile dressing over the access site and further anchor the pacing catheter with tape to prevent accidental dislodgment.

10. Following implantation, obtain a chest roentgenogram to check proper positioning of the pacing catheter and confirm that a pneumothorax has not developed during placement. Ideally, obtain both AP and lateral chest roentgenograms to check for lead positioning. An AP chest roentgenogram by itself cannot confirm proper positioning of the pacing catheter.

B. SEQUENTIAL ATRIOVENTRICULAR PACING

Equipment
In addition to the equipment needed for transvenous ventricular pacing, you will need the following.

1. Atrial pacing catheter (either a or b).
   a. A separate atrial pacing catheter to be used in conjunction with a ventricular pacing catheter, as described above. An atrial J wire is best, as

the curve of this wire allows for the most stable positioning of the catheter against the atrial wall.
  b. A combination catheter with both ventricular and atrial components.
2. A pulse generator (either a or b).
  a. An external pulse generator capable of functioning in a DVI mode (paces both the atrium and ventricle, senses only the ventricle, and is inhibited only by a sensed ventricular event).
  b. A bipolar dual-chamber pacemaker. Special connections are required for this type of pacemaker.

Required Monitoring

As for ventricular pacing.

Required Laboratory Data

As for ventricular pacing.

SEQUENTIAL ARTERIOVENTRICULAR PACING PROCEDURE

Depending on whether one or two pacing catheters are to be inserted, one or two venous access sites are required.

1. Set up the equipment as described earlier for ventricular pacing.
2. Although placement of an atrial catheter can be performed with electrocardiographic guidance, ideally, it should be done with fluoroscopic guidance.
  a. Fluoroscopic guidance.
    (1) Atrial J wire.
      (a) Advance the atrial J wire through the venous access sheath into the atrium.
      (b) Turn the curve of the wire medially and slowly withdraw the catheter until the tip

catches on the atrial appendage. Look for a rocking motion of the catheter in the appendage parallel to the AV groove that confirms the catheter is positioned in the atrial appendage.

   (c) Although the atrial appendage is the most stable site for temporary atrial pacing, if you fail after several attempts to position the catheter in the right atrial appendage, position the atrial J wire on the lateral wall of the atrium.

 (2) Combination atrial and ventricular catheter.

   (a) Advance the combination catheter into the venous sheath.

   (b) Position the right ventricular lead in the ventricular apex, as discussed earlier. Then position the atrial lead in the right atrium, preferably in the right atrial appendage.

b. Electrocardiographic guidance.

 (1) Atrial J lead.

   (a) Advance the atrial J catheter through the venous sheath.

   (b) Connect the distal electrode to the V lead of the EKG machine.

   (c) Advance the catheter further into the right atrium with EKG monitoring. Electrograms will appear as in Figure 25–2,A and B and Figure 25–4,A.

   (d) Turn the catheter so the J loop faces medially. (Use the marker outside the body for directional information).

   (e) Pull the catheter back slowly until contact is made with the atrial myocardium as evidenced by PR segment elevation in the electrogram (Fig 25–4,B).

 (2) Combination atrial and ventricular catheter.

   (a) Advance the combination catheter through the venous sheath.

   (b) Attach the distal electrode of the ventricular pacing catheter to the V lead

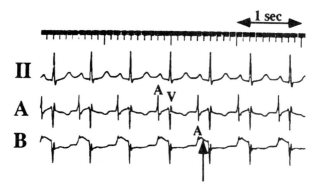

FIG 25–4.
Simultaneous recordings of surface electrocardiographic *lead II* and intra-cardiac unipolar recordings from the right atrial cavity *(A)* and the right atrial endocardial surface *(B)*. Note the PR segment elevation *(arrow)* that occurs when the catheter is up against the atrial endocardium. These two recordings were both made in the right atrial appendage. A = atrial depolarization; V = ventricular depolarization.

of the electrocardiograph.
  (c) Position the ventricular lead by electrocardiographic monitoring, as described earlier.
  (d) Once the ventricular lead is in place, attach the distal electrode of the atrial pacing catheter to the V lead of the electrocardiograph.
  (e) Position the atrial pacing catheter in the atrium as described previously.
3. Confirm adequate pacing function. Because in most situations the pulse generator to be used functions in the DVI mode, only atrial capture or pacing threshold must be confirmed.
  a. Measurement of atrial capture threshold is sometimes made difficult by the relatively low amplitude P waves that are noted on the monitoring leads. For this reason, examine multiple EKG leads for evaluation of atrial capture. If AV conduction is intact, atrial capture can be confirmed by an associated increase in the ventricular rate.

b. To determine the atrial pacing threshold, set the pulse generator to a rate significantly faster (usually 10 to 20 beats/min) than the patient's intrinsic atrial rate. If the patient does not require ventricular pacing during atrial threshold testing, turn the ventricular output down to a minimum. Set the atrial output to a minimum value and slowly increase current output until atrial capture is noted. This current is the atrial pacing threshold. Ideally, the pacing threshold should be less than 2 mamp. To provide an adequate safety margin, set the pacing output at 2 to 3 times the threshold value.

In general, when treating a patient with AV sequential pacing, adjust the atrial and ventricular outputs. Based on the determined thresholds, adjust the ventricular sensitivity and rate as clinically indicated and adjust the AV delay to achieve optimal hemodynamic benefit.

FOLLOW-UP

1. Keep the patient at complete bed rest for at least 24 hours.
2. Examine the insertion site daily for evidence of infection. Note any tenderness, erythema, swelling, or drainage of pus.
3. Confirm adequate pacing function daily in the following manner.
   a. Check whether the patient has a stable underlying heart rhythm by slowly decreasing the pacing rate by 5 to 10 beats per minute with the patient in the supine position. The pacing rate may be turned as low as 30 beats per minute to allow for recovery of slow ventricular escape rhythms. **Never abruptly turn off the pacemaker if the patient is being paced.**

b. If the patient is symptomatic, check the pacing threshold only, as described.

c. If the patient is asymptomatic at the slow rates and has a stable rhythm, check both pacing and sensing thresholds, as described.

d. Both pacing and sensing thresholds may vary from day to day, especially if treatment with new antiarrhythmic agents is initiated. Adjust the pulse generator to appropriate settings.

4. To evaluate the patient's response to therapy, obtain a 12-lead EKG during pacing and compare it with the tracings obtained during pacing catheter placement. Similarly, record the unipolar and bipolar electrograms from the pacing catheter and compare with the initial tracings.

COMPLICATIONS

See Chapter 2 for discussion of complications of central venous access. Specific complications related to the temporary pacing system are as follows.

1. *Infection.* If the pacing site appears infected, remove the pacing catheter and the venous sheath as soon as possible and obtain bacterial cultures. Depending on the degree of infection and the clinical situation, antibiotic treatment may be indicated for a variable length of time.

2. *Perforation of the right ventricular wall.* The patient may have symptoms of pleuritic chest pain or may be asymptomatic. A pericardial friction rub may be heard. Suspect this complication if a change in the electrogram recorded from the pacing catheter develops. Figure 25–5 shows an electrogram recorded from the distal tip of the pacing catheter that may be indicative of penetration of the pacing catheter beyond the endocardium. Compare this electrogram with that shown in Figure 25–2,D. Variation from the baseline recording of the 12-lead

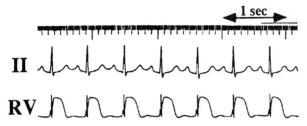

FIG 25–5.
Simultaneous recordings of surface electrocardiographic *lead II* and intracardiac unipolar recordings from the right ventricular wall. Note the predominant R wave in the right ventricular recording and the marked ST
segment elevation.

electrocardiogram during pacing also may indicate
perforation. If perforation is suspected, withdraw
the catheter; if indicated, place a fresh catheter.
Generally, perforations seal spontaneously without
significant complications. However, particularly in
patients who are anticoagulated, bleeding into the
pericardium may occur and, rarely, lead to
pericardial tamponade requiring pericardiocentesis.
When perforation is suspected in anticoagulated
patients, it is recommended that anticoagulation be
stopped, if possible.
3. *Arrhythmias.* Ventricular arrhythmias including
premature ventricular complexes, ventricular
tachycardia, and ventricular fibrillation may
develop during pacing catheter insertion.
Arrhythmias are more likely to occur in patients
with acute myocardial infarctions. Although, pacing
may precipitate ventricular arrhythmias, it is less
likely once the catheter is in a stable position.
Catheter dislodgement may lead to ventricular
arrhythmias. Therefore, continuous EKG
monitoring of patients with temporary pacing
catheters is required. If new ventricular
arrhythmias appear after pacing catheter
placement, check catheter position by evaluation of
a paced 12-lead EKG (compare with baseline EKG)
and a chest roentgenogram. You may have to
reposition the pacing catheter.

4. *Pacemaker malfunction.* Generally, two types of pacing problems can occur: failure of sensing, or capture. If pacemaker malfunction is suspected, first check all the connections from the pacing catheter to the connecting cables and from the cables to the pulse generator. If the battery was not changed recently, install a new battery in the pulse generator. If a component malfunction in the pulse generator is suspected, change the pulse generator; however, pulse generator malfunction is rare.

a. Capture failure is diagnosed when a pacing stimulus applied when the ventricle is not refractory does not result in capture of the ventricle. For example, a pacing stimulus delivered in the ST segment of a native QRST complex (due to poor sensing of the complex) would not be considered failure to capture because the ventricle is probably refractory at this time. When failure to capture is diagnosed, recheck the pacing threshold. If an acceptable pacing threshold is obtained, appropriately adjust the output of the pulse generator. Usually no further manipulations are required. However, if the pacing threshold is unacceptably high and all the connections are intact, you may need to reposition the catheter. Fracture of the pacing catheter may also lead to inappropriately high pacing thresholds or inability to pace. Switching to a unipolar pacing system may avert this problem.

b. Failure to sense. Two types of sensing failure may occur:

(1) Oversensing will cause false inhibition of the pacemaker output. This is diagnosed with documentation of heart rates below the set pacing rate. Sometimes the signal that is oversensed can be easily detected on a monitor strip recording. Place a set of calipers, opened to the programmed pacing interval, with the right end of the calipers on

the pacing stimulus, and observe where the left end falls. If it falls on the T wave, this may indicate oversensing of T waves. Remember it does not have to fall on the peak of the T wave on the monitor strip because the intracardiac tracing will look different than the monitor tracing. Sometimes it will not be obvious on the monitor strip what is causing the oversensing. If oversensing is a problem, check the sensing threshold and adjust the sensitivity so that the sense light blinks only once for each native QRS complex.

(2) Undersensing is diagnosed when the pulse generator generates a pacing stimulus when it should have been inhibited by the patient's intrinsic rhythm or a premature ventricular contraction. If undersensing is suspected, check the sensing threshold and adjust the sensitivity appropriately. When the sensitivity is set to its minimum value, undersensing should not be a problem.

A pacing catheter fracture may also lead to sensing problems. If adjusting the sensitivity does not correct the problem, attempt to continue utilizing the pacing system by switching it from a bipolar system to a unipolar system.

Procedure to Switch From a Bipolar to a Unipolar System

The temporary pacing system is designed to be a bipolar system. However, should a sensing or pacing problem occur that cannot be corrected by the techniques already described, switch the pacing system to function as a unipolar pacing system. The unipolar electrogram may be larger than the bipolar electrogram, which may allow for improved sensing. Changing the pacing system to unipolar function might resolve an undersensing problem. If failure to pace is the problem, check each of the electrodes for electrical continuity. To do this, connect the surface leads of the EKG machine to the patient as previously described and connecting the V lead to each of the proximal and distal pacing catheter electrodes sequentially. Record intracardiac unipolar electrograms. Each electrode should record an intracardiac potential as shown in Figure 25–2. If an intracardiac electrogram is not obtained, a problem with that electrode may be present. If the distal pacing catheter electrode is functional, convert the pacing system to unipolar function as follows.

1. Insert the distal electrode back into the negative position in the pulse generator and apply insulating tape over the positive electrode.

2. Apply a surface electrode to the skin and connect to the positive output port of the pulse generator.

3. Check pacing and sensing thresholds as described.

DOCUMENTATION

Following placement of a temporary venous pacing system, write and sign a procedure note in the progress notes of the patient's chart. The note must include the following.

1. Indication for temporary pacing.

2. Type of pacing (transvenous ventricular pacing or sequential atrioventricular pacing).

3. Choice of site of venous cannulation.

4. Size and types of pacing catheters used.

5. Technique used for positioning of catheters (fluoroscopy versus electrocardiographic monitoring).

6. Complications encountered, if any.

7. Pacing and sensing threshold data.

8. Strips of unipolar and bipolar recordings made, if any.

9. Analysis of 12-lead paced EKG output, including bundle branch morphology and axis.

10. Programmed settings, including rate, pacing output in milliamperes, and sensitivity setting.

11. Postprocedure chest roentgenogram documenting the presence or absence of a pneumothorax and position of the pacing catheter.

While the transvenous pacemaker is in place, the following should be documented in the chart daily.

1. Pacing and sensing thresholds, if they can be safely obtained.

2. Analysis of a 12-lead paced EKG.

3. Presence or absence of escape or underlying rhythm, if this can be safely performed.

4. Programmed settings including rate, pacing output in milliamperes, and sensitivity setting.

SUGGESTED READING

Bing OHL et al: Pacemaker placement by electrocardiographic monitoring, *N Engl J Med* 287:651, 1972.

Holmes DR Jr: Temporary cardiac pacing. In Furman S, Hayes DL, Holmes DR, editors: *A practice of cardiac pacing*, New York, 1989, Futura, p 209.

Syverud S: Cardiac pacing, *Emerg Med Clin North Am* 6:197, 1988.

Wharton JM, Goldschlager N: Temporary cardiac pacing. In Saksena S, Goldschlager N, editors: *Electrical therapy for cardiac arrhythmias*, Philadelphia, 1990, WB Saunders, p 107.

26

External Transcutaneous Pacing

Jeffrey Goldberger, M.D.
Alan Kadish, M.D.

INTRODUCTION

Transvenous pacing is one of the most reliable modes of temporary pacing. However, it does require an invasive procedure. It requires time to insert a properly functioning transvenous pacemaker. Transcutaneous pacing can be achieved more quickly than transvenous pacing. It is, therefore, appropriate as first line therapy in patients requiring emergency pacing. It may also be used as a back-up in situations where the chances that pacing will be required are small and the benefits of transvenous pacing do not outweigh the risks. The major disadvantages of transcutaneous pacing are

1. It is not as reliable as transvenous pacing.
2. It is usually uncomfortable for the patient because the current needed to achieve successful pacing is generally high.

OBJECTIVE

Successfully pace the heart with a transcutaneous pacing system.

Indications

1. Emergency pacing.
2. Back-up in situations in which the chances that pacing will be required are small.

Contraindications

None.

PREPARATION

Equipment

1. External pacing electrodes.
2. External sensing electrodes (may be the same as pacing electrodes).
3. External pacemaker.

Required Monitoring

None.

Required Laboratory Data

None.

PROCEDURE

1. Apply the pacing and sensing electrodes to the patient according to the manufacturer's instructions.
2. If the patient is asystolic, set the pacemaker to maximal output to attempt to capture the ventricle.
3. If the patient has an underlying cardiac rhythm,

display the electrocardiogram (EKG) on the external pacemaker unit. Set the gain to adjust the size of the EKG so that it is appropriately sensed.

4. To determine the capture threshold, set the pacemaker rate faster than the patient's intrinsic rate. Turn the pacemaker on at the lowest output setting and slowly increase the output until ventricular capture is achieved.

5. Set the output only slightly higher than the capture threshold to minimize patient discomfort.

6. If adequate pacing thresholds cannot be obtained or the patient is having too much discomfort, slightly adjust the pacing electrode position.

FOLLOW-UP

Once adequate external transcutaneous pacing is achieved, decide whether the patient needs continuous or back-up pacing. If continuous pacing is required, proceed with placement of a transvenous pacemaker as outlined in Chapter 25. If the patient only requires back-up pacing, turn the external pacemaker rate below the patient's intrinsic rate.

COMPLICATIONS

Short-term use of an external transcutaneous pacemaker can be tolerated by a large percentage of patients and is associated with relatively few complications. However, the following potential problems may arise.

1. *Difficulty with assessment of capture.* The most critical aspect of temporary pacing is successful capture and pacing of the ventricles. Because external

transcutaneous pacing utilizes pulse widths of 20 to 40 ms (compared to 2 ms for transvenous pacing) and current outputs ranging from 40 mamp to 200 mamp (compared to less than 5 mamp for usual transvenous pacing), the pacing output may obscure the QRS complex resulting from depolarization of the ventricles. Many of the monitoring systems that come with the external pacemakers have special built-in circuitry that results in a blanking period for a short time following the pacing stimulus to allow for better visualization of the paced QRS complex. However, assessment of capture by EKG monitoring may still be difficult.

Adequacy of capture can be inferred from demonstration of restoration of effective circulatory function. External transcutaneous pacing can result in significant skeletal muscle contraction that might make determinations of the presence or absence of a carotid or radial arterial pulse difficult. Palpating the femoral artery provides the best method to determine the presence or absence of an adequate pulse. The most reliable assessment of successful ventricular pacing is an improvement in the patient's mental status. Successful ventricular capture is confirmed if a patient, previously obtunded due to poor cardiac output secondary to bradycardia, subsequently wakes up when external transcutaneous pacing is initiated.

2. *Patient discomfort.* External pacing may result in skeletal muscle contraction and cutaneous nerve stimulation, both of which may lead to patient discomfort and pain. Patient discomfort does not necessarily correlate with the level of current used. Treatment with analgesics or benzodiazepines may be required in order to continue transcutaneous pacing.

3. *Skin irritation.* Under the pacing electrodes, skin irritation is generally not a problem, especially when pacing is performed for a short period of time. However, prolonged transcutaneous pacing can lead to skin irritation and breakdown.

DOCUMENTATION

After treatment with external transcutaneous pacing, write and sign a procedure note in the patient's chart that includes the following:

1. Indication for temporary pacing.
2. Whether external pacing was successful and the pacing threshold that was used.
3. Whether the patient tolerated external pacing.
4. Treatment plan regarding future temporary pacing for the patient, for example, temporary transvenous cardiac pacing or continued back-up pacing with the external pacing system.

SUGGESTED READING

Holmes DR Jr: Temporary cardiac pacing. In Furman S, Hayes DL, Holmes DR, editors: *A practice of cardiac pacing*, New York, 1989, Futura.

Syverud S: Cardiac pacing, *Emerg Med Clin North Am* 6:197, 1988.

Wharton JM, Goldschlager N: Temporary cardiac pacing. In Saksena S, Goldschlager N, editors: *Electrical therapy for cardiac arrhythmias*, Philadelphia, 1990, WB Saunders.

27

Transthoracic Cardiac Pacing

Thomas G. Frolich, M.D.

INTRODUCTION

Emergency cardiac pacing may restore electrical and thereby mechanical activity during asystolic cardiac arrest, although it is unlikely to improve the dismal prognosis of this condition. The ready availability of transvenous pacing (see Chapter 25) and recent improvements in techniques for transcutaneous pacing (see Chapter 26) have diminished the need for emergency transthoracic pacing. Transthoracic pacing, a relatively simple technique, remains useful in situations where other methods of pacing are not available.

OBJECTIVE

To pace the heart during asystolic cardiac arrest using a transthoracic pacing electrode.

Indications

1. Asystolic cardiac arrest when *all* of the following conditions are met.
   a. Drug treatment with atropine (at least 1.0 mg) and epinephrine (high dose, 5.0 mg) has failed to restore an effective rhythm.
   b. Transcutaneous pacing has been unsuccessful or is not available.
   c. Rapid placement of a transvenous pacing electrode is not possible.
2. Severe bradycardia (less than 20 beats/min) accompanied by hemodynamic collapse when *all* of the following conditions are met.
   a. Progressive rapid hemodynamic deterioration in spite of all medical supportive measures, including administration of oxygen; ventilatory support; rapid intravenous fluid infusion; placement of the patient in Trendelenburg position; and administration of atropine, isoproterenol, and vasopressors.
   b. Transcutaneous pacing has been unsuccessful or is not available.
   c. Rapid placement of a transvenous pacing electrode is not possible.

Contraindications

1. A patient with cardiac function that is stable or can be stabilized with medical treatment.
2. Ready availability of transcutaneous or transvenous pacing.
3. Cardiac arrest with electromechanical dissociation, a circumstance in which cardiac pacing is of no benefit.
4. Ventricular fibrillation, a circumstance in which cardiac pacing is of no benefit.

Prolonged cardiopulmonary arrest (longer than 20 minutes) is a relative contraindication. Cardiac pacing is extremely unlikely to be of value.

PREPARATION

Asystolic cardiac arrest carries a worse prognosis than does arrest from ventricular fibrillation. The probability of successful resuscitation depends on the duration of the asystole. Emergency pacing is most likely to be of benefit if instituted within the first few minutes after cardiopulmonary arrest. It is almost never useful as a final desperate measure, when instituted 15 or more minutes after the onset of cardiac arrest.

Equipment

1. Transthoracic pacing kit. Two different types of kits are currently available.
   a. Trocar type. A kit would include the following.
      (1) Transthoracic placement needle, consisting of a 15 cm long, 18-gauge, blunt cannula with a solid 17 cm long sharp inner obturator.
      (2) A 34 cm long bipolar pacing wire stylet with a preformed J-shaped distal tip and a 10-cm space between the proximal and distal electrodes.
      (3) An electrical adaptor, which connects the pacing stylet and pulse generator.
   b. Hollow-needle type (Fig 27–1). A kit would include the following.
      (1) A 13 cm long, thin-walled, 17-gauge transthoracic placement needle with a sharp beveled tip.
      (2) A pacing stylet, similar to the one used in the trocar type kit, preloaded in the placement needle, with its proximal end extending out of a side port through an adjustable hemostatic valve.
      (3) A 10-mL syringe.
      (4) An electrical adaptor to attach the pacing stylet to a pulse generator.
2. Portable demand pulse generator.
3. Antiseptic solution.

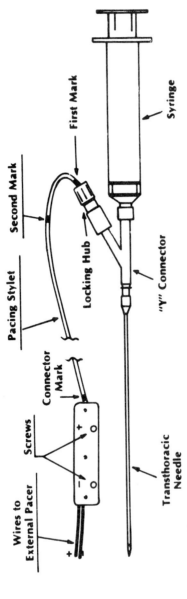

FIG 27–1.
The *transthoracic needle, Y connector, syringe, pacing stylet* and *electrical connector.* Note the first and second marks on the pacing stylet, which are used to position the stylet in the ventricle, and the connector mark, which is used to place the electrical connector properly on the stylet.

4. Sterile 10-mL syringe.
5. Sterile gloves.
6. Suture and/or tape to secure pacing stylet and pulse generator to the patient.
7. The following items are useful, but not essential; the procedure should not be delayed because of their immediate unavailability.
   a. A basin filled with sterile solution (water or saline) for injection.
   b. Sterile towels.

Required Monitoring

Electrocardiography is required. The limb leads should be left connected to the patient to allow continuous observation of cardiac rhythm during pacemaker placement.

Required Laboratory Data

None.

PROCEDURE

The pacing stylet may be introduced by either the subxiphoid or parasternal approach. The subxiphoid approach usually results in right ventricular placement; left ventricular placement is more likely with the parasternal approach. The subxiphoid approach is preferred. However, if the introducer needle cannot be positioned properly with a subxiphoid approach, the parasternal approach should be used.

Subxiphoid Approach

With its bevel up, insert the placement needle in the left xiphocostal notch, 1 cm to the left of the xiphoid tip and 1 cm below the costal margin, and direct the needle toward the midpoint of the left clavicle, at an angle

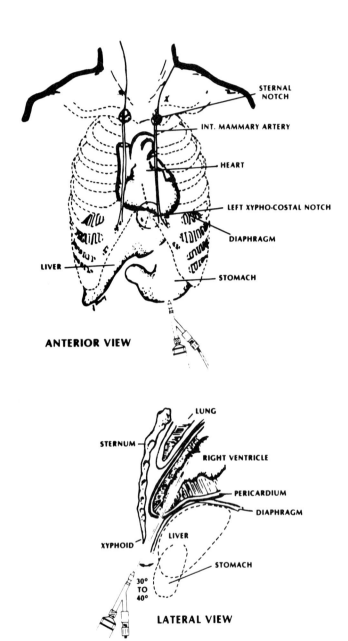

FIG 27–2.
Diagram showing subxiphoid approach for introduction of the placement needle. The needle is inserted at the left xiphocostal notch and directed toward the sternal notch. Insert the needle at an angle of between 30° to 40° to the skin.

of 30° to 40° to the skin. (Fig 27–2). The risk of laceration of the left lobe of the liver is increased if the needle
is introduced at a more perpendicular angle to the skin.
If this approach fails, attempt placement again with
the needle directed cephalad toward the sternal notch,
at an angle of 30° to 40° to the skin.

Parasternal Approach

Insert the needle in the fifth intercostal space, just
lateral to the left sternal border and direct medially,
dorsally, and cephalad, toward the right second costo-
chondral junction at an angle of 30° to the skin.

Place the pacing stylet as follows:

1. Verify proper EKG connection and that the cardiac
   rhythm requires emergency pacing.
2. Put on mask and sterile gloves.
3. Clean the skin around the xiphocostal notch
   (subxiphoid approach) or the left fifth intercostal
   space at the parasternal border (parasternal
   approach) with an iodophor solution.
4. Allow the lungs to passively deflate.
5. Interrupt cardiopulmonary resuscitation (CPR)
   during introducer needle placement. It should be
   possible to resume CPR within 30 seconds; if
   placement is unsuccessful, CPR must be resumed
   before another attempt is made. The techniques for
   pacing stylet placement are slightly different for
   trocar and hollow-needle pacing kits.
   a. Trocar type.
      (1) Advance the plastic straightener to the
          distal end of the pacing stylet to straighten
          the J curve. Place the stylet on a sterile
          towel.
      (2) While firmly holding the sharp inner
          obturator against the hub of the blunt
          cannula, advance this assembly toward the
          heart, using either the subxiphoid or
          parasternal approach already described. The

cannula should be advanced about 8 to 10 cm, depending on the size of the patient.

(3) Remove the inner obturator and immediately connect the 10-mL syringe.

(4) Attempt to aspirate blood. If blood return is obtained, proceed with pacing stylet insertion. If blood return is not obtained, withdraw the cannula while exerting constant negative pressure on the syringe. Resume CPR before making any further attempts at pacemaker placement.

(5) Once blood return is obtained, remove the syringe and insert the straightened tip of the pacing stylet into the placement cannula.

(6) Advance the pacing stylet and remove the plastic straightener. When the stylet is advanced beyond 17 cm, the J-tip will emerge from the cannula and reform within the ventricular cavity. It may be possible to feel this transition; if not, advance the stylet until only 8 to 10 cm extends beyond the hub of the needle, or until firm resistance is met. To avoid the possibility of shearing off the J-tip, once the tip has been advanced beyond the end of the cannula, the stylet should not be withdrawn back through the cannula.

(7) While stabilizing the stylet's position relative to the heart, withdraw the introducer cannula and slide it off the proximal end of the pacing stylet.

(8) Resume CPR.

(9) Slide the electrical adaptor over the end of the pacing stylet, making sure the stylet is pushed all the way into the hole in the adaptor. Secure the adaptor by tightening the thumb screws and attach the positive and negative connectors to the corresponding terminals of the pulse generator.

(10) Set the pulse generator as follows.
   (a) Rate at 80 cycles/min.
   (b) Output at maximum (usually 20 mamp).
   (c) Sensitivity on asynchronous (or turn the dial all the way toward the highest millivolt setting.)
(11) Turn the pulse generator on.
(12) Interrupt CPR and observe the EKG for evidence of ventricular capture. Pacing spikes should be present regardless of capture; to confirm capture, look for the presence of a QRS complex **and a T-wave** following the pacer spike. A carotid or femoral pulse should be checked as evidence of mechanical as well as electrical activity.
   (a) If pacer spikes are present without evidence of capture, gently manipulate the position of the pacing stylet. Initially, advance the stylet; if capture does not result, slowly withdraw the stylet. If capture is still not obtained, resume CPR, withdraw the pacing stylet completely, and reattempt pacing stylet placement.
   (b) If pacer spikes are not visible, resume CPR; check the connections and the pulse generator. Most generators have a light or needle gauge that indicates when the unit is generating a pulse. If this indicator does not show pulse activity, the pulse generator may have a depleted battery or may be defective.
(13) Once ventricular capture is achieved, secure the pacing stylet to the chest wall by suture or tape. Tape the pulse generator to the patient. If appropriate, the pulse generator settings may then be adjusted to provide for demand pacing.
(14) Obtain a six-lead (or 12-lead, if available) EKG to document capture.
(15) Obtain a chest roentgenogram and examine

for evidence of pneumothorax and proper pacing stylet position.

(16) Because the stability of electrical capture is not assured with a transthoracic pacing stylet, place a temporary transvenous pacemaker as soon as possible (see Chapter 25).

b. Hollow-needle type.

(1) Verify the proper positioning of the preloaded pacing stylet within the introducer needle. The first of two black marks on the stylet should be just visible outside the hemostatic valve prior to insertion.

(2) Tighten the hemostatic valve by rotating it clockwise.

(3) If immediately available, withdraw sterile water or saline through the injector needle into the attached syringe. Expel all air from the syringe and needle.

(4) Advance the introducer needle assembly through the skin toward the heart, using either the subxiphoid or the parasternal approach. Once the needle tip has punctured the skin, apply constant negative pressure with the syringe and rapidly advance the needle until blood return is obtained.

(5) Once blood return is observed, if indicated, inject epinephrine or calcium chloride into the heart. If rapid blood return is not obtained, withdraw the needle with constant negative suction and resume CPR before further attempts at pacemaker placement are made.

(6) Once blood return is obtained (with or without subsequent intracardiac injection), insert the pacing stylet. Stabilize the introducer needle, loosen the hemostatic valve, and advance the pacing stylet until

the second black mark is aligned with the valve. In this position, the distal "J" curve of the stylet will have exited the needle and reformed within the ventricle.

(7) To maintain the stylet position within the ventricle, advance the stylet further through the hemostatic valve while the introducer needle is withdrawn. Slide the needle completely off the pacing stylet and attach the electrical adaptor.

(8) Proceed with cardiac pacing as described above [Steps 5,a,(10) through 5,a,(16)].

FOLLOW-UP

1. Determine and correct, if possible, the underlying cause of the cardiac rhythm disturbance. If continued pacing is indicated, the patient should be moved as little as possible until a transvenous pacing lead is positioned and functioning properly.

2. When transthoracic pacing is no longer required, remove the stylet with gentle traction on the proximal end. Apply an antiseptic ointment and small bandage over the insertion site.

COMPLICATIONS

An accurate assessment of complications of emergency transthoracic pacing is not possible. The scant clinical data relating to this procedure, and the corresponding data relating to intracardiac injections, suggest that complications are rarely of clinical significance.

1. *Cardiac tamponade.* Although hemopericardium appears to be fairly common following intracardiac injection and transthoracic pacemaker placement, the incidence of tamponade is very low.

2. *Coronary artery laceration.* The subxiphoid approach avoids the major epicardial vessels, usually allowing one to enter the right ventricle on its diaphragmatic surface. Recent studies suggest that the parasternal approach, as described, rarely causes coronary injury.

3. *Pneumothorax.* Careful attention to proper anatomic landmarks minimizes the risk of this complication. Examination of the chest roentgenogram and auscultation of the lungs following successful resuscitation is essential to detect this potential complication.

4. *Laceration of other organs.* Lung, liver, gastric, and great vessel lacerations are possible but of unclear clinical significance.

DOCUMENTATION

Upon completion of the procedure, write a Transthoracic Pacemaker Placement note in the progress notes of the patient's chart. The following information should be included.

1. Indication for emergency transthoracic pacing, including clinical and hemodynamic data, pertinent rhythm strips, and a description of the medical measures taken prior to pacemaker insertion.

2. Technique employed (subxiphoid or parasternal approach) and number of insertion attempts.

3. If successful pacing was achieved, include pacemaker settings (milliamperes, rate, and sensitivity), with a rhythm strip demonstrating ventricular capture.

4. Clinical status of the patient following the procedure.

5. Any complications recognized during the procedure.

6. Findings of follow-up chest auscultation and roentgenogram.

SUGGESTED READING

Roberts JR: Emergency transthoracic cardiac pacing. In Roberts JR, Hedges JR, editors: *Clinical procedures in emergency medicine,* Philadelphia, 1991, WB Saunders.

Tintinalli JE, White BC: Transthoracic pacing during CPR, *Ann Emerg Med* 10:113, 1981.

28

Intra-Aortic Balloon Pump

Carl L. Tommaso, M.D.

INTRODUCTION

The intra-aortic balloon pump (IABP) has become the mechanical device most commonly used for circulatory support. It is extremely effective. Because of the large-bore balloon and the sophisticated nature of insertion and management, trained and experienced personnel are necessary for its safe application.

OBJECTIVE

To support left ventricular function with an IABP.

Indications

1. Cardiogenic shock.
2. Heart failure refractory to pharmacologic treatment.
3. Unstable angina refractory to pharmacologic treatment.

4. Mechanical complications of myocardial infarction, (for example, ventricular septal rupture, papillary muscle rupture, or dysfunction).

5. Intractable ventricular tachycardia resulting from myocardial ischemia or causing hemodynamic instability.

6. Cardiac support for high-risk patients undergoing non-cardiac surgery.

7. Reversible septic shock causing severe hemodynamic impairment.

8. Difficulty in weaning a patient from cardiopulmonary bypass.

9. Support and stabilization during high-risk coronary arteriography or angioplasty.

Contraindications

1. Severe aortic insufficiency.

2. Abdominal aortic aneurysm.

3. Severe obstructive aortic, aorto-iliac, or peripheral vascular disease.

4. Severe bleeding diathesis (may preclude percutaneous insertion).

PREPARATION

Because IABPs require a large-caliber catheter to be inserted through the femoral artery, it is important to assess the vascular system of the patient's lower extremities prior to insertion. If possible, the use of non-invasive studies such as Doppler pressures is advisable; however, the luxury of such assessment is frequently not available. Evaluation of the arteries of the lower extremities with contrast material injection during coronary arteriography or prior to angioplasty may be performed to identify the presence of obstructive lesions or severe arterial tortuosity that may interfere with the advancement of the balloon pump catheter. However, given the circumstances under which most IABPs are inserted, thorough and careful palpation; recording of the femoral, popliteal, dorsalis pedis, and posterior tibial pulses; and auscultation over the femoral arteries are frequently the only examinations that can be done.

Either femoral artery can be used for insertion. The right iliofemoral system usually has less angulation at the aortic bifurcation than does the left and under most circumstances is the preferred site of introduction. However, other variables—such as the need for coronary angiography or angioplasty, prior use of the right femoral artery for an invasive procedure or the presence of vascular disease—may make the left femoral artery a preferred site.

Intra-aortic balloon pump insertion is best accomplished in a coronary care unit or cardiac catheterization laboratory. The presence of fluoroscopy is extremely helpful, though not mandatory.

Equipment

1. Intra-aortic balloon pump.
2. An IABP catheter. Several different parameters need to be considered when choosing an IABP catheter for a patient. These include the following.
   a. *Balloon volume.* Balloon volumes range from 30 to 60 mL. A 40-mL balloon is usually used, but the size may have to be adjusted upward or downward depending on patient size.
   b. *Central lumen.* The IABP catheters come either with or without a central lumen. A guidewire, passed through the central lumen, facilitates placement, particularly in tortuous vessels. After the guidewire is removed, this lumen can be used to monitor aortic pressure. Attempted passage of the catheter without a guidewire increases the risk of dissection of the iliofemoral vessels or aorta.
   c. *Balloon shaft size.* Depending on the manufacturer, balloon catheters have an 8.5 F to 12.0 F shaft size. Usually the 8.5 F and 9.5 F

catheters do not have a central lumen. The 10.5 F and larger sizes incorporate a central lumen.

3. Equipment required for intra-aortic balloon insertion.
   a. Angiographic needle set.
   b. Two guidewires. The central lumen of a balloon catheter will accommodate only a 0.03-inch guidewire, while the dilator and sheath introduction are best accomplished over a 0.035-inch or 0.038-inch guidewire.
   c. An 8 F dilator.
   d. An introducer sheath, appropriately sized for the balloon catheter to be used, preferably with a hemostatic valve and matching introducer sheath dilator.
   e. A three-way stopcock.
   f. A 60-mL syringe.
   g. A one-way valve.
   h. Connector tubing.
   i. Pressure monitoring set (for pressure measurement through the central lumen).
   j. Basin of sterile 0.9N saline.
   k. Local anesthetic (such as lidocaine, 1%).
   l. Scalpel blade.

Required Monitoring

1. Electrocardiographic monitoring, with connections to a monitor that can be seen by the operator and also to the IABP console, for timing and monitoring.

2. Intra-arterial pressure monitoring, either through a peripheral artery (see Chapter 1) or through the central lumen of the IABP catheter.

Required Laboratory Data

1. Prothrombin time, partial thromboplastin time, complete blood count, and platelet count.

2. Chest roentgenogram to ascertain and document appropriate positioning following insertion.

PROCEDURE

1. Sheath insertion.
   a. Select the insertion site. The site should be approximately 2 cm below the inguinal ligament.
   b. Prepare the site in usual manner. Shave the hair in the patient's groin area and cleanse the skin with topical antiseptic.
   c. Administer local anesthesia with lidocaine 1% or 2%. Raise a skin weal with a 25-gauge needle; then infiltrate on each side of the artery, using a 20- or 21-gauge needle. To avoid intra-arterial injection of local anesthesia apply suction with the barrel of the syringe during infiltration.
   d. Insert an angiographic needle into the femoral artery. A brisk return of pulsatile, oxygenated blood should be appreciated. If the patient is in shock, the blood return may not be pulsatile, nor may it look oxygenated, and entry into a vein must be considered. The best way to differentiate artery from vein is to insert a guidewire and check the course of the vessel under fluoroscopy.
   e. To facilitate passage of the dilator and sheath, insert a 0.035- or 0.038-inch guidewire through the needle and pass it smoothly through the ilio-femoral system to the aorta, under fluoroscopic guidance, if available. If there is resistance to passage of the wire, do not push; resistance usually signals that the guidewire is not appropriately placed.
   f. Nick the skin with a scalpel at the site of insertion to facilitate passage of the dilator and sheath.
   g. Remove the needle, but leave the guidewire in place.
   h. Pass an 8 F dilator over the wire to dilate the skin and vessel wall.
   i. Remove the dilator, but leave the guidewire in place and apply pressure over the puncture site

to control bleeding. Wipe the guidewire clean.
j. Advance the sheath and dilator set over the guidewire. Leave about 1 inch of the sheath exposed outside the skin. A hemostasis valve on the sheath is not necessary, but is helpful. The dilator and guidewire can be left in the sheath while the balloon is being readied, or they can be removed and the sheath capped with the stopcock if a hemostatic valve is not provided with the sheath. If an 0.030-inch wire is used to insert the sheath, it can be left in place and the readied IABP catheter backloaded on to it for insertion.
2. Prepare the IABP catheter.
   a. Follow the manufacturer's instructions. Usually the balloon is prepared while still in the sterile packing tray.
   b. Attach the one-way valve to the catheter and apply 30 to 60 mL of negative volume, with a large syringe.
   c. Remove the catheter from the tray.
   d. If the balloon has a central lumen and is to be inserted over a wire, remove the stylet and flush the central lumen of the catheter with sterile saline. If other than a 0.030-inch wire was used for sheath insertion, preload the catheter with a 0.030-inch wire.
   e. If fluoroscopy is unavailable, measure the length of balloon to be inserted by holding the distal end of the balloon at the angle of Louis or between the second and third intercostal space, and measure the distance down to the umbilicus and obliquely to the insertion site. Mark or note the position of the proximal end of the balloon catheter at the skin line.
3. Insertion of the IABP catheter.
   a. Remove the introducer dilator and wire (if larger than 0.030 inch). If a hemostatic valve is present, no significant blood leakage should occur; however, if there is no hemostatic valve on the

sheath, a torrential amount of bleeding can occur and the sheath must be pinched at its shaft, where it extends beyond the skin.

b. Insert the distal end of the balloon into the sheath over the guidewire and advance 5 to 10 cm beyond the distal tip of the IABP catheter. Then advance the balloon and guidewire, as a unit, under fluoroscopic guidance.

c. Advance the catheter until the radiopaque marker on the distal tip of the catheter lies about 2 cm distal to the origin of the left subclavian artery.

d. If a 0.030-inch guidewire was used for sheath insertion and left in place, backload the IABP balloon and advance to appropriate position.

e. If fluoroscopy is unavailable, advance the catheter until the skin line mark (see 2e) reaches the skin.

f. If during insertion the patient complains of pain in the groin or back, dissection of the aorta or ilio-femoral system may have occurred (See Complications).

g. Once the catheter is placed, withdraw the sheath until no more than 5 inches remain within the femoral vessel, to ensure that the entire balloon has exited the sheath.

h. Remove the guidewire, and aspirate blood through the central lumen. Then connect the central lumen to a standard, calibrated pressure monitoring line.

i. Release the vacuum by removing the one-way valve. On some catheter models it is necessary to rotate a knob on the distal end of the balloon to "unwrap" the balloon. On most models, initiation of pumping will inflate the balloon. Pumping should be initiated as soon as possible to avoid the development of thrombi on the balloon.

j. If fluoroscopy was not used for insertion, obtain a roentgenogram and review as soon as possible to confirm the catheter position.

k. Once proper balloon position is confirmed and the balloon is functioning normally, fit the sheath seal (which comes in place over the shaft of the balloon), over the sheath and suture the seal to the skin.

l. Caveats to be Remembered.

(1) When possible use fluoroscopy.

(2) Do not use excessive force. This may result in tearing or dissection of the artery or damage to the balloon.

(3) The guidewire or stylet must be in place in the central lumen during balloon insertion.

(4) If fluoroscopy is not used, an immediate roentgenogram is necessary after balloon placement.

(5) The IABP will not operate if any part of the balloon is still within the sheath; therefore, the sheath must be pulled back.

(6) Do not inject air or drugs into the central lumen (iodinated contrast material may be injected under fluoroscopy to assess position).

4. Initiation of IABP.

A person familiar with the operation of an IABP must be available to initiate and operate the IABP console. Each console has individual operating instructions that must be followed.

a. Connect the balloon catheter to the console by means of a sterile connecting tubing.

b. Initiate (fill) the balloon according to the console manufacturer's instructions.

c. Set the timing of the balloon inflation and deflation. Balloon inflation and deflation timing can be set to the arterial pressure wave or the EKG.

(1) Pressure wave timing. Timing can be guided by the arterial pressure wave form from either the central lumen of the IABP catheter or a separate arterial line (Fig 28–1). The IABP unit should be timed so that the balloon inflates at the dicrotic notch of the aortic pressure wave tracing and deflates just

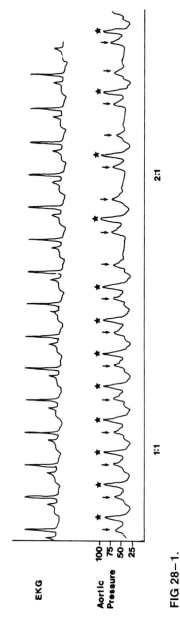

FIG 28–1.

Diagram showing electrocardiographic tracing and simultaneously recorded aortic pressure tracing. The strip shows counter-pulsation at a 1:1 and a 2:1 ratio. *Arrows* indicate nonaugmented pulsation; *stars* indicate augmented pulsation.

prior to the onset of systole (opening of the aortic valve). Optimum timing will cause a slight reduction in the systolic pressure of the beat following augmentation and a 10 mm Hg to 15 mm Hg presystolic dip below the nonaugmented diastolic pressure.

If the wave form from the central lumen is not used for timing, but timing is done from another peripheral arterial site, then compensation for pulse transmission to site of the intra-arterial line (50 ms) must be made.

(2) Electrocardiographic timing. Some units can be timed from the EKG tracing, with inflation timed to the T wave and deflation to the P wave.

d. It is recommended to begin balloon inflation at 1:2 (one inflation for every other heartbeat) while adjusting the timing. Instructions for timing are contained in the operating manual of the IABP console.

Timing of the balloon is critical and must be done by an experienced person. Incorrect timing can result in systole occurring while the balloon is inflated, which may lead to a disastrous outcome, particularly in critically ill patients.

Irregularity of cardiac rhythm (atrial fibrillation or frequent ectopic beats) leads to difficulty in timing the balloon, and alterations in timing or management of the arrhythmia may be necessary.

FOLLOW -UP

1. Check the IABP functioning, observing the pressure wave form to ensure that the appropriate wave form is present. Fluoroscopic viewing of the balloon to ensure that it is opening fully is helpful.

2. Once the balloon is inserted, institute anticoagulation. Heparin is the anticoagulant most commonly used for this purpose.

3. During balloon use, the platelet count may fall. Check the platelet count daily.

4. Check the groin daily for evidence of infection, bleeding, and hematoma throughout the time the balloon catheter is in place.

5. Check the distal pulses manually, or by Doppler, daily to ensure adequate perfusion of the lower extremity.

6. Maintain the patient supine or up to 30° head up while the balloon is in place.

Balloon Catheter Removal

There is no maximum time that a IABP catheter can be left in place; however, the longer the catheter is in place, the more likely are the development of infectious and thrombotic complications. The risk of these complications must be balanced against the patient's need for the device and the risks of removal and reinsertion of the catheter at another site.

1. Prior to removal of the IABP, ascertain that the patient's cardiac output is not dependent on the IABP. To assess dependency, sequentially reduce the counterpulsation frequency from 1:1 to lower frequencies (the lower frequencies are programmed on the console by the manufacturer), and observe cardiac performance for several hours to ensure stability.

2. Once it is decided that the IABP can be removed, halt the anticoagulation (heparin) 3 hours prior to removal of the catheter.

3. Disconnect the catheter from the console and attach a large syringe (50 mL or greater) to the inflation lumen of the catheter. Apply negative pressure with the syringe to fully deflate the balloon.

4. Release the skin sutures or other means of securing the catheter, and remove the balloon and sheath as

a unit. After inflation, the balloon is larger than the sheath; therefore, it should not be withdrawn into the sheath, but the catheter and sheath removed together. Failure to do this may result in shearing of the balloon and embolization of balloon fragments to the lower extremity. If difficulty or undue resistance is encountered when the catheter is removed, there may be thrombus formation around the balloon, and removal by arteriotomy may be indicated. If the patient has a bleeding diathesis, surgical repair of the artery may be necessary after the catheter is removed.

5. Compress the femoral artery below the site of puncture as the balloon is being withdrawn, to prevent distal embolization. Allow the artery to bleed for several beats. Then compress the artery proximally and allow back-bleeding for several beats.

6. Compress the puncture site and maintain compression until the bleeding ceases, usually 30 to 60 minutes. Pressure may be maintained manually or by use of a compression device.

7. Observe adequacy of distal limb perfusion during and after artery compression. If there is inadequate perfusion, obtain vascular surgical consultation.

COMPLICATIONS

1. Balloon membrane rupture or perforation can occur during IABP counterpulsation. It can be caused by membrane fatigue or contact with a sharp instrument or calcified plaque during insertion. Perforation is usually gradual, though large gas emboli have been reported. It is usually signaled by an alarm on the console or the appearance of blood in the catheter tubing. If perforation occurs, do the following.
   a. Stop the pumping.
   b. Remove the catheter (as described earlier).
   c. Consider placing the patient in the Trendelenburg position.

2. During or after removal, limb ischemia may occur as a result of thrombosis or emboli. This will be signaled by pain, loss of warmth and color, and mottling of the affected extremity. Treatment includes the continuation of heparin and obtaining prompt vascular surgical consultation. Catheter removal may be necessary.

3. Aortic dissection during insertion of the catheter may occur. Dissection is signaled by severe pain in the patient's groin or back during insertion. Dissection can be confirmed with fluoroscopy by the injection of a small amount of contrast material through the central lumen of the catheter. If dissection has occurred, vascular surgical consultation should be obtained, the balloon and sheath removed, and the patient monitored for evidence of vascular obstruction or inadequate limb perfusion. Another site must be used for insertion.

4. With prolonged insertion, infection can occur. Usual attention to indwelling lines and aseptic techniques during insertion and care is necessary.

5. Renal failure has been noted as a result of IABP. Monitoring of renal function on a daily basis is necessary.

6. Thrombocytopenia has occurred during IABP use. Monitoring by complete blood count and platelet counts on a daily basis is warranted.

DOCUMENTATION

On completion of catheter insertion, write an IABP Insertion note. This must include

1. Indication for IABP counterpulsation.
2. Site of catheter insertion.
3. Catheter type and size used.
4. Complications encountered, if any.
5. Documentation of placement by chest roentgenogram or fluoroscopy.

SUGGESTED READING

Aroesty JM: Percutaneous intra-aortic balloon insertion. In Grossman W, editor: *Cardiac catheterization and angiography,* ed 3, Philadelphia, 1986. Lea & Febiger.

Serota H et al: High risk cardiac catheterization. In Kern M, editor: *The cardiac catheterization handbook,* St Louis, 1991. Mosby–Year Book.

29

Percutaneously Inserted Cardiopulmonary Bypass

Carl L. Tommaso, M.D.

INTRODUCTION

Percutaneously inserted cardiopulmonary bypass (PCPB) has recently become available at most major medical centers for use in short-term circulatory support.

The PCPB procedure utilizes large-caliber vascular cannulae, inserted percutaneously or by cut-down, most commonly into the femoral vessels. Deoxygenated blood is removed from the right atrium under negative pressure, pumped through a heat exchanger and membrane oxygenator, and then returned to the body via the femoral artery and retrograde aortic flow. Figure 29–1 is a schematic representation of a PCPB system.

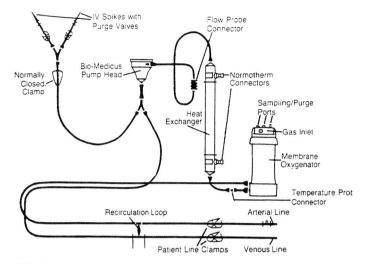

FIG 29–1.
Schematic diagram of the components of a percutaneously inserted cardiopulmonary bypass system.

OBJECTIVE

Short-term support of cardiopulmonary function by means of a percutaneously placed cardiopulmonary bypass.

Indications

Use of PCPB may be indicated in patients who need short-term cardiac and/or pulmonary support for a number of reasons, including

1. Cardiogenic shock.
2. Cardiac arrest.
3. Heart failure following cardiac surgery.
4. Drug overdose.
5. Acute pulmonary insufficiency.
6. High altitude pulmonary edema.
7. Hypothermia.
8. Failed interventional cardiac procedures.

9. Prophylactic assistance, in patients undergoing high-risk procedures.

10. Mechanical complications of myocardial infarction prior to cardiac catheterization and surgery.

Contraindications

1. Severe aortic insufficiency.
2. Abdominal aortic aneurysm.
3. Severe obstructive aortic, aorto-iliac, or peripheral vascular disease.
4. Severe bleeding diathesis.

PREPARATION

Similar to the preparation for the insertion of the intra-aortic balloon pump (IABP) (see Chapter 28). The vasculature of the lower extremities must be evaluated by clinical, noninvasive, or angiographic means.

Required Personnel

The cannulae are relatively easy to insert either percutaneously or by surgical cut-down. If a cut-down is employed, it should be performed by either a surgeon or a cardiologist skilled in the procedure for femoral vessel cutdown. For percutaneous insertion, any physician experienced in vascular invasive procedures can easily insert the cannulae.

Although the pump is quite simple to operate, it does require a trained perfusionist. Hence, in addition to the usual catheterization support staff, a perfusionist must assist with the procedure. Availability of a cardiac anesthesiologist during the time the patient is on PCPB adds to the safety of its use.

Equipment

The PCPB system has several components including the vascular cannulae and connecting tubing in series with a flow probe, a heat exchanger, a membrane oxygenator, and the console.

1. Vascular cannulae.
   a. The venous cannula, 16 to 20 F, is inserted over a tapered dilator. The cannula plus the connections is 75 cm in length. It contains 34 sideholes in addition to a large endhole. It is inserted through a femoral vein and positioned with the cannula tip in the right atrium.
   b. The arterial sheath and connector are 32 cm in length and 16 to 20 F in caliber. The apparatus has 14 sideholes and also is inserted over a tapered dilator.

2. The connecting tubing. The connector on the arterial sheath is termed "female"; the connector on the venous cannula is termed "male." The tubing has appropriate reciprocal connectors.

The tubes that connect the cannulae to the extracorporeal console are clear plastic ⅜-inch polyvinyl chloride lines. These lines include a recirculation loop and clamps to occlude the lines. The lines are connected to the pumphead and pump to form a closed system. The circuit incorporates separate lines to prime the apparatus.

3. The pumphead is of a conical shape and rotates to form a vortex, which pumps the blood with minimal damage to the cellular components.

Equipment Required for PCPB Insertion

1. Angiographic needle set.
2. Stiff guidewires, 0.035 or 0.038-inch in diameter.
3. Dilators 8, 12, and 14 F.
4. Local anesthetic (lidocaine 1% to 2%).
5. Scalpel blade.

Required Monitoring

Insertion for PCPB is accomplished best in a coronary care unit, operating room, or cardiac catheterization laboratory. The presence of fluoroscopy is extremely helpful, though not mandatory for placement of the venous cannula. The following are required.

1. Electrocardiographic monitoring that can be seen by the operator.
2. Intra-arterial pressure monitoring.
3. Pulmonary artery pressure monitoring.

Required Laboratory Data

1. Prothrombin time and partial thromboplastin time.
2. A complete blood count and platelet count.
3. A chest roentgenogram to ascertain and document appropriate positioning of cannulae is required following insertion.

PROCEDURE

1. Insertion of vascular cannulae.
   a. The site and technique for PCPB insertion is similar to that of the IABP (see Chapter 28). However, both arterial and venous access is required.
   b. Prepare the site for percutaneous catheter insertion in the usual manner; shave the skin and cleanse the area with an antiseptic solution.
   c. Administer local anesthesia (see Chapter 28).
   d. Attach an angiographic needle to a syringe and insert it into the femoral vein while maintaining negative pressure on the syringe until a free-flowing return of nonoxygenated blood is appreciated.
   e. Insert a stiff 0.035 or 0.038-inch guidewire through the needle and advance it smoothly through the femoral vein to the inferior vena cava and right atrium under fluoroscopic control, when available. If resistance to the

passage of the wire is encountered do not push against resistance; resistance usually signals that the guidewire is not placed appropriately.

f. Make a small nick with the scalpel in the skin at the site of insertion to facilitate passage of the dilator and cannula.

g. Remove the needle but leave the guidewire in place.

h. Sequentially pass the 8, 12, and 14 F dilators over the guidewire to dilate the percutaneous tract and vessel wall.

i. While applying pressure at the puncture site to control bleeding, remove the dilator but leave the guidewire in place. Wipe the guidewire clean.

j. Advance the cannula and dilator set over the guidewire until the distal end is positioned in the midportion of the right atrium. Then remove the dilator and guidewire and rapidly close the clamp on the cannula.

2. Arterial cannula insertion.

a. Insert an angiographic needle into the femoral artery; a brisk return of pulsatile oxygenated blood will be noted. If the patient is in shock, the blood return may not be pulsatile, nor look oxygenated, and possible entry into a vein must be considered.

b. The arterial cannula is inserted in the same manner as described for the venous cannula.

c. Advance the arterial cannula into the iliofemoral system.

3. Connection to the pump.

a. Administer heparin, 300 units/kg, before beginning bypass.

b. Have the perfusionist fill the connecting tubing with saline. All air must be removed from the connecting tubing before the tubing is connected to the vascular cannulae.

c. Attach the cannulae to the saline-filled, air-purged, connecting tubing.

d. After verifying that the tubing is free of air, open the clamps and start the pump.

FOLLOW-UP

The PCPB should only be used a short period of time; hence, the follow-up of the device is limited to the time it is in place and must be done by the operator and perfusionist. The PCBP procedure provides in excess of 5 L/min of cardiopulmonary bypass, which should be adequate to perfuse all organ systems provided the patient has a normal metabolic rate. However, perfusion may not be adequate in situations of increased metabolic demand that require increased blood flow, such as trauma, anemia, sepsis.

Because of nonpulsatile flow during bypass, vasodilation occurs, resulting in the marked warmth and perspiration that patients often experience. Pulmonary artery, PAOP, and systemic pressures often drop markedly because of the unloading nature of the pump and the vasodilation. It is recommended that mean systemic blood pressures be kept in the range of 60 to 70 mm Hg to maintain perfusion of the coronary vessels and other organ systems. Use of short-acting alpha-agonists, for example, phenylephrine, and volume replacement may be necessary to maintain systemic blood pressure.

Unlike the cardiopulmonary bypass systems used in the cardiac operating room, the PCPB system does not vent the left ventricle. Because relatively small catheters are used to drain the right atrium, pulmonary blood flow might still exist and left ventricular distention could result.

Because blood is removed from the right atrium with negative pressure, there is a possibility of significant air embolism. Therefore, venous lines and insertion sites must be meticulously watched.

Attention to the insertion site for signs of bleeding, thrombosis, infection, skin necrosis, and nerve palsy is required.

Removal of PCPB

1. Before removal of the PCPB, ascertain that the patient's cardiopulmonary function is not dependent on PCPB. Decrease the flow rate through the pump and observe cardiovascular function. If the patient remains hemodynamically stable it is appropriate to discontinue PCPB.

2. The cannulae can be removed either surgically and the vessels repaired under direct vision, or they can be removed percutaneously, in a manner similar to the method described for the IABP (see Chapter 28). Because of the required administration of large doses of heparin and the large bore of the catheters, there is a real danger of hematoma formation. Maintain pressure over the insertion site manually or with a compression device.

3. Observe the adequacy of distal limb perfusion during and after artery compression. If there is inadequate perfusion, obtain vascular surgical consultation.

COMPLICATIONS

1. Vascular insufficiency. Because of the large bore of the arterial cannula, vascular insufficiency and its sequel are common problems. If the cannula was inserted through a cut-down, a distal perfusion line from the arterial line may be inserted into the femoral artery for distal perfusion. Following removal of the arterial cannula, femoral artery thrombosis can develop and contribute to vascular insufficiency.

2. Air embolization. The venous drainage is achieved with negative pressure created by the pump. Therefore, insertion of the cannula and any other venous lines and insertion sites must be air tight.

3. Insertion site bleeding and hematoma formation after cannulae removal.

4. Infection at the insertion site.

DOCUMENTATION

Upon completion of the procedure write a note in the chart that includes:

1. Indication for PCPB.
2. Site of vascular cannulations.
3. Size of cannulae inserted.
4. PCPB pump flowrate.
5. Heparin dosage given and subsequent anticoagulation regimen to be followed.
6. Any complications encountered during initiation of PCPB.

SUGGESTED READING

Overlie P: Emergency use of portable cardiopulmonary bypass, *Cathet Cardiovasc Diagn* 20:27–31, 1990.

Shawl FA et al: Percutaneous cardiopulmonary bypass support in high-risk patients undergoing percutaneous transluminal coronary angioplasty, *Am Heart J* 64:1258–1263, 1989.

Tommaso CL: Use of percutaneously inserted cardiopulmonary bypass in the cardiac catheterization laboratory, *Cathet Cardiovasc Diagn* 20:32–38, 1990.

Index

C